DIABETES
MELLITUS

DIABETES MELLITUS

and

Human Trafficking

Kenneth W. Shipman

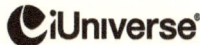

**Diabetes Mellitus
and Human Trafficking**

iUniverse books may be ordered through booksellers or by contacting:

*iUniverse
1663 Liberty Drive
Bloomington, IN 47403
www.iuniverse.com
1-800-Authors (1-800-288-4677)*

*ISBN: 978-1-4917-6087-1 (sc)
ISBN: 978-1-4917-6088-8 (e)*

Print information available on the last page.

iUniverse rev. date: 02/18/2015

The author has made every attempt as a researcher to provide credit to every source used for this publication. I want to especially that Dr. Richard K. Bernstein for his books and radio broadcasts and Dr. Albert Bandura, professor at Stanford University who emailed me pointing me toward his work chapter by chapter several years ago on his social cognitive theory. Also Dr. Phillip Raskin, the Chair of Biomedicine at the University of Southwestern Medical Center for allowing me to be a participant in his research on aldose reductase inhibitors in the 1990's and his advice concerning the Parkland Hospital's Diabetes Clinic. There are many others who I have made every attempt to credit in this publication. I apologize if I have left anyone out but any notification through the publisher will be corrected immediately. My purpose is to invite others to promote awareness about diabetes and early detection, diabetes literacy and management and to also create awareness about health needs among those that may be victims of human trafficking.

Kenneth W. Shipman

I would like to share with you some of my personal experiences managing diabetes and listening to people who have suffered in Laos and Thailand that were victims of human trafficking and were diabetic. When I first was told I had diabetes I didn't know what to think but soon discovered that injecting insulin and eating was a part-time job requiring a skill I didn't. There was a learning curve and as I approach senior living am discovering there is a new learning curve.

Advice and literature was overwhelming and I thought each one was correct until I made up my mind that I must choose what worked for me. My relationship with the endocrinologist was important and I had to change a few times. In addition there were new products brought to market promising to provide better control but I think it was better profit.

Those persons living in Asia I met were not as lucky as they had to go for long periods of time with no treatment, no diet considerations or knowledge of what was wrong with their bodies. If you are interested in this you may search the Internet as copyright laws prohibit me writing about those pieces of literature.

When I was diagnosed with diabetes I was given a blood glucose meter and told to check my blood glucose often and attempt to balance the readings on the meter between 80 and 100. A dietician talked to me but nothing she said worked. If I took too much insulin I had to eat something to keep from passing out and if I didn't take enough insulin I had a number more than 120 and was chastised for it with more instructions. I am sharing my experience not the experience of others. However, I did feel sorry for those involved in human trafficking taken from their home of origin and made to work with no care.

There was a stigma for me of having diabetes at first and then I didn't care. However, there is still discrimination. Initially people would tell me about their families that lost a leg or legs or went blind. They tell these things without any consideration of the diabetic and don't realize they might be scaring the person. Some people would feel it their duty to ask about your health in a tone of mighty concern. This said not knowing they would die within several years and I am still here.

Doctor after doctor would proclaim that a cure was just around the corner 45 years ago and none has come yet. The drug companies make a lot of money selling diabetic supplies for people, cats, dogs and what else? But there is nothing about them taking the initiative in helping those captured and traded in human trafficking.

Insulin is the medicine I inject each day but copyright law prevents me from writing about its discovery and history but you can easily look this up on the Internet. This I feel is the greatest time in history to have diabetes. Also if you are interested in helping organizations that are helping those caught in the throes of human trafficking you can find those on the Internet also and may wish to help.

Table of Contents

Chapter 1 Sugar on the Brain. The brain weighs approximately three pounds, looks like tofu, has innumerable neuronal connections and is well supplied with blood. If blood sugar falls too low the body or brain goes into a coma and may be fatal. This low blood sugar is called severe hypoglycemia. What happens when blood sugar is too high or hyperglycemia? At some point unique to the individual blood sugar that is too high can cause vomiting, convulsions, lethargy and difficulty breathing to name a few of the symptoms. High blood sugar too can be fatal. The human brain processes information best when blood sugar is within the parameters of normal or controlled within normal.

I have been living with diabetes over forty years and take insulin, observe a diet that works best for me, and exercise). It is important to understand that it's up to you to take control of your diabetes. You may have to fire your doctor. Does it shock you to know that most diabetics are non-compliant with recommended blood sugar levels and average blood sugar levels and do not follow their doctor's directions? Physicians cannot provide optimal care if diabetics ignore their instructions for medication and diet.

Your choice is this, you take control of the diabetes and accept the damage or you take charge of your diabetes and accept the benefits. It is not easy, it's tedious sometimes, some diabetic's burnout but you can do it and it's worth it. What do you have against you? Burnout The concept of the term "burnout" was attributed to psychologist Herbert J. Freudenberger in 1975. The phenomenon while in the dictionary was not applied to self-help groups, addicts and others with chronic illnesses (Freudenberger, 1975). Hans Selye refers to distress, experienced that is excessive and demanding that causes harm to the body, and eustress, which is positive for the body contributing to happiness and health (Selye, 1978).

In professional settings among leaders burnout usually begins about one year after a person starts a new job. This concept can also be applied to other workers as well as chronic illness such as diabetes mellitus.

Managing diabetes mellitus is a part-time job. Most of the information about diabetics and the management of the disease mention briefly the difficulty in managing and living with the chronicity of the disorder, there is a paucity of literature labeling the illness as potentially contributing to "burnout" because of the time, and attention to detail required to successfully live with the disorder. The stress of managing the disease can lead to burnout and in turn depression, suicide, divorce and no friends. This is evident in the literature (Lundman, Asplund, & Norberg, 1988). A diabetic has to live a very organized life in order to maintain a metabolic balance that contributes to both physical and mental health. Stress from managing the daily blood tests and visits to a health practitioner often results in "unrelieved stress" (Lundman, Asplund, & Norberg, 1988).

How does Diabetes Mellitus reduce the speed of action potential in the pancreas, cell, and the brain? Insulin-dependent diabetes is when the pancreas cannot secrete enough insulin, and requires regular insulin injections. Non-insulin-dependent diabetes is when the pancreas does secrete insulin but neither the liver or muscle cells respond properly to it, and usually begins relatively late in life and is associated with obesity. When blood sugar is too high blood glucose levels rise and stay high.

It is clear that the brain has the ability in sensing the levels of glucose. Glucosensing neurons are clearly a distinct class of metabolic sensors with the capacity to respond to a variety stimuli. This makes it likely that these glucosensing neurons do involve energy balance and the regulation of glucose levels. This neuron specifically has the ability to sense, and regulate energy homeostasis in the body. However, when the body is out of control with a disease technology and self-management are necessary. (Dwyer, 2002)

Motivation and a goal are also essential if good health is an achievement. This study is about how many longitudinal studies and some persons I interviewed manage diabetes mellitus. Unfortunately, even with the gift of insulin and scientific studies of applying self-management most diabetics do not choose to manage their. Diabetes correctly and maintain a healthy blood sugar. Do diabetics need to go to meetings like Alcoholics Anonymous? Does America or the World need Diabetics Anonymous? Sugar is made by humans, so is alcohol.

A little sugar may cause a craving for too much or an uncontrollable appetite for daily industrial doses of sugar. I have watched persons eat an entire box of chocolate covered cherries. Ask yourself, is that unhealthy? The lack of research about health literacy and self-management of diabetes from the perspective of the diabetic makes it difficult for people suffering from this chronic illness to make illness-management decisions. The purpose of this research is to look for themes in self-management that reveal possible pathways for diabetics to discover how to self-manage diabetes and improve health-literacy.

The actual attitudes and experiences of diabetics will contribute to the body of knowledge to solve this research problem. There are over 28 million Web sites, thousands of books, and millions of pages on Google listing the word diabetes and the complications of diabetes. All of this information can be confusing for people with diabetes and limited health literacy. The goal of this researcher is to learn about health-literacy and the self-management of diabetes from the perspective of the diabetic, to provide qualitative evidence that the health-literacy with skillful self-management behavior is a commodity of self-efficacy that cannot be purchased.

Using thematic analysis in a generic, qualitative inquiry, the researcher will examine viewpoints, thoughts, and reflections, to understand diabetes self-management. Table of Contents CHAPTER 1. INTRODUCTION 2 CHAPTER 2. LITERATURE REVIEW 8 CHAPTER 3. METHODOLOG 30 CHAPTER 4.

DATA COLLECTION AND ANALYSIS 76 CHAPTER 5. CONCLUSION 148 REFERENCES 169 CHAPTER 1. INTRODUCTION Introduction to the Problem When people are diagnosed with diabetes mellitus (DM or diabetes), their pancreases may produce some insulin. Eventually, however, insulin production ceases. The timing of this event varies among diabetics.

For some people with diabetes, adaptive behaviors, such as eating a good diet and following an exercise plan, including appropriate weight control, reverses the need for insulin or oral diabetic medications forever (Bernstein, 2003; 2007). For others, dietary control and exercise are helpful, at first, to manage the disease. However, some people cannot maintain the appropriate levels of intensity in management and must seek new avenues of self-management. In all cases, the intent is to remain in glycemic control that does not cause diabetic complications.

The key strategy to maintaining control of DM is to develop and encourage self-efficacy in adhering to a diabetes regimen. The goals of the ADA are to fight for those affected and against the deadly consequences of diabetes. They do this by teaching proactive coping skills and planning strategies, and arranging personal support systems for people with diabetes. These goals lead to improved physical and psychological healing.

The quality of life is synergistically related to health-literacy and self-management choices (Arkowitz, Westra, Miller, & Rollnick, 2007; Atkins, 2004; Bernstein, 2007; O'Neill, Westman, & Bernstein, 2003). Background of the Study Diabetes is physiologically complex in the human body. These complexities are challenges to the psychological and intellectual states of the person with DM. The most important issues patients have found in dealing with DM are knowledge of the disease, quality of life, anxiety, and depression. These issues change the lives and lifestyles of people and their families. It appears that the best way to deal with these issues is to become proactive in managing diabetes.

Both collecting information about the diabetes and record keeping are essential for optimum physical and psychological health. The patient's personal beliefs, perceptions, and attitudes about diabetic control are the keys to achieving normal blood sugar levels. Questionnaires and tests are valuable instruments for doctors and other health professionals to use to collect information to educate and propose a treatment for a diabetic to follow (Davidson, 2000). But this is only the beginning. The intensity of self-management challenges the capacities of the diabetic. Self-management of diet, exercise, and medication, even for a short period, may become stressful.

Research indicates that increasing motivation and reducing ambivalence toward change arouses intrinsic desires for people with diabetes choosing to improve the quality of their lives (American Diabetes Association [ADA], 2007; Creer, 1997). The effectiveness of diabetic education may necessarily include an intervention by family members or professional health-care providers. Interventions are used to gain the attention of non-compliant diabetics. An attempt to empower the diabetic to own responsibility for his or her self-care results in positive lifestyle habits that contribute to health benefits and potential survival. The significance of self-regulation and self-efficacy to accomplish positive results is supported by research (McCaul, Glasgow, & Schafer, 1987), crossing all socio-economic, racial, and psychological variables.

Historically, lower income groups have been more non-compliant and have less-than-favorable access to positive health care when diabetes education is required. The disease may be exacerbated by unhealthy eating habits and lack of physical activity (Kavanaugh, Gooley, & Wilson, 1993). Statement of the Problem People with diabetes mellitus experience health-literacy and self-management problems from the first days of diagnosis. As the tedium of detail and the continuous responsibility for well-being are realized, the self-efficacy of the individual is challenged (Polonsky, 1999).

In addition, an exhaustion of physical, mental, and emotional strength may eventually impair motivation to self-manage this chronic illness. Stress often results from the continuing challenges required for successful management of the disease (Sperry, 2008). Management decisions are stressful as the diabetic strives to balance medication, diet, and exercise in order to reduce co-morbidities, complications, and end-stage progression. Because of the stresses involved, many diabetics suffer psychologically for years before experiencing the physical complications of the disease.

More people die yearly from diabetes than from breast cancer and AIDS together (ADA, 2010). Diabetes management products, and their illusion of hope for living with diabetes, are not matched with the challenge of integrating health-literacy and self-management skills (Polonsky, 1999). Purpose of the Study This research has three related purposes. The first purpose is to identify qualitatively, utilizing a generic-qualitative method, how people with diabetes mellitus acquire health-literacy. The second purpose is to determine how self-management expertise is learned.

The final purpose is to collect generic-qualitative information on how to improve the process. Rationale This study is needed to articulate the urgency of improving how people with diabetes live with the illness. Although not as grievous today, diabetes once meant limited lifestyle, unemployment, isolation, and certain death. The general population is not aware of the difficulty of facing life with that kind of label. Persons with a chronic illness have lost something once taken for granted, their good health. The experiences of people diagnosed with diabetes mellitus can provide insights about courageous living and creativity in the battle against their disease.

They, along with their experiences, can best provide the insights needed for resolution. Fear and outdated phobias are not useful for learning to self-manage diabetes. They have reinvented themselves, defeated fear, maintained spiritual hope, and are winning against their condition. This researcher is approaching the topic of self-management with the belief that there are always new answers. Keeping up to date with the cutting edge of research is of the utmost importance to the diabetic. New information is necessary for change to occur.

The resulting information will be useful for psychologists who work with people with diabetes; motivation for the patients and information for both the patients and the therapists is vital. Healthcare professionals are taught how to diagnosis DM, but not how to teach self-management of the condition. Diabetes educators are educated about management systems, but not about techniques leading to adequate self-management. There is no compendium of information for psychologists in dealing with people with diabetes. This study will enable psychologists to assist those patients to learn about health literacy or find information about their condition. Currently, the empowerment of self-efficacy is not a priority. Change in this area is needed because diabetes is a serious disease.

Diabetes is a disease of blame and shame, with physicians who do not suffer from the disorder crying non-compliance while they manage the disease in the most cost effective manner possible. Diabetics are accused of non-compliance, mismanagement, and cheating on diets. Diabetic complications involve not only people who hide from the realities of the disease, but people who are managing the disease, also (Bernstein, 2007; Bradley, 1994; Falvo, 2004). People who are doing well with diabetes are congratulated and respected for their ability to control their disease.

They become the people used in advertisements: the happy face, and not the burden of disease beneath, endorses the philosophy of tolerating, rather than curing, diabetes. For policy makers, philanthropists, employers, and the public to feel compelled to discover a way to cure diabetes, they must understand that diabetes is costly for society. The costs to society are rising and pervasive. The incidence of the disease is accelerating, and the effects of the disease are extremely damaging. There is no cure. Diabetes is one of the worlds oldest, deadliest, and most insidious of diseases (Sperry, 2008). Not every diabetic has health insurance, access to healthcare, or knows how to get help from public charities or welfare agencies.

Although many educational programs are extremely successful, they are not necessarily available for the low literate, the poor, and those with limited access to information. Syringes, insulin, and testing equipment are expensive. The United States is not addressing this disease realistically for the poor and the illiterate. Treatment in the third world is even worse (Bradley, 1994; Guthrie & Guthrie, 2008). Definitions of Terms Blood glucose. This is the main sugar found in the blood and is the body's main source of energy. It is also referred to as blood sugar.

This is the amount of glucose in a given amount of blood. It is noted in milligrams in a deciliter, or mg/dL. Blood glucose monitoring. This refers to checking blood glucose levels on a regular basis. Its primary purpose is to enable the management of diabetes. A blood glucose meter (or blood glucose test strips that change color when touched by a blood sample) is needed for frequent blood glucose monitoring. Complications. Complications include all the harmful effects of diabetes, such as damage to the eyes, heart, blood vessels, nervous system, teeth and gums, feet and skin, or kidneys.

Glucose is one of the simplest forms of sugar. It is used by the body for energy (ADA, 2007). Insulin. Insulin is a hormone that helps the body use glucose for energy. When the body cannot make enough insulin, it is taken by injection or through use of an insulin pump (ADA, 2007). Insulin-dependent diabetes mellitus (IDDM). This is the former term for Type 1 diabetes (ADA, 2007). Motivational interviewing.

"Motivational interviewing is a collaborative, person-centered form of guiding to elicit and strengthen motivation for change" (Miller & Rollnick, 2009, p. 137). Self-management. In diabetes, this refers to the ongoing process of managing diabetes. Self-management includes meal planning, planned physical activity, blood glucose monitoring, taking diabetes medicines, and handling episodes of illness and of low and high blood glucose, managing diabetes when traveling, and more. The person with diabetes designs his or her own self-management treatment plan in consultation with a variety of health care professionals such as doctors, nurses, dietitians, pharmacists, and others (ADA, 2007). Team management.

The researcher is seeking to talk to approximately 10 people, but there are no limitations about the kind of person who will be invited or volunteer to participate. Research utilizing thematic analysis provides rigor, themes, and patterns in relation to epistemological and ontological positions that are useful and flexible (Kostere & Percy, 2006). Self-management of diabetes is not assumed to be science or certain, or the last word in understanding the self-management of diabetes (Popper, 1986). Thematic analysis provides an approach to methodological data with rigor. It offers the researcher an opportunity to be explicit and clear about what the researcher is doing.

Thematic analysis requires that attempts are in accordance with the proposal. It is a good fit for the qualitative research of diabetes mellitus and self-management because the researcher may write with balance and consistency for the epistemological intent of the study (Kostere & Percy, 2006). There is the possibility that an inexperienced researcher may not analyze the data at all. There exists a temptation to use the interview questions as themes in explaining the data, instead of analyzing it. Analysis of the data will not be simple.

It will require much work in order to present a convincing analysis, deriving and supporting each theme with appropriate material from the collection and presenting it in a format that may be adequately understood by the reader (Kostere & Percy, 2006). The collection and processing of recorded data from participants relate to hard-to-control-for, yet potentially potent, confounding variables or factors that could be the true hidden causes of what this researcher thinks was observed. Things may have happen during the interview and analysis process, but not necessarily for the reasons the researcher thinks they did.

Issues of credibility, believability, or internal validity of the findings and results impact and limit the researcher's ability to process everything with 100% accuracy. Generic Qualitative Inquiry Generic qualitative inquiry is useful for the purpose of this research to produce the greatest clarity about the self-management of diabetes from the perspective of the diabetic. Qualitative research uses reflections, thoughts, opinions, attitudes, and beliefs willingly shared, without the shaping influence of the researcher. Themes from the transcribed material of the research will be discovered.

They will be acquired from thinking critically about the self-reporting techniques and self-management capacities of the diabetes participants. In discussing their individual processes of self-management, participants with diabetes mellitus will give voice to previously unacknowledged pieces of the story of diabetes. Therefore, the researcher will be active in seeking the themes and seeking a critical position (Braun & Clarke, 2006). The design of this study on self-management of diabetes is grounded in the theory of self-regulation based on social cognitive theory (Bandura, 1986).

Social learning of self-regulatory skills is in the hands of the diabetic, rather than the physician (Bandura, 1986). Diabetics cannot change their health habits by willpower, alone. The quality of diabetic health requires using motivational and self-management skills. This concept is a paradigm shift, from treating diabetics in the disease model to treating them in the health model. By adopting goals as a guide to the work required to realize and maintain health, a social and cognitive engagement is more than biomedical management (Bandura, 2005).

Building on the model of Bandura's self-management of Asthma study and publication (1986), this research is an attempt to contribute to learning about diabetes self-management progressing in small steps to enhance self-efficacy (Bandura, 2005). Albert Bandura's (1986) social cognitive theory is an explanation of human adaptability and the intrinsic perception of personal behavior, environment, and cognition to survive with a chronic disease.

This researcher proposes the literature from the past 90 years is indicative of the difficulties encountered when managing insulin dependent diabetes mellitus (Banting, 1922; Galmer, 2008; Guthrie & Guthrie, 2008; Tattersall, 2009). Organization of the Remainder of the Study The remainder of this proposal is organized into two additional chapters: first, the review of the literature for the study; then the methodology used for the study. CHAPTER 2. LITERATURE REVIEW Introduction This literature review focuses on the available research about the genealogy of a diabetic person's perspective of the self-management of diabetes mellitus.

How do subjective opinions, attitudes, beliefs, reflections of experiences, and self-management of insulin dependent diabetes mellitus (IDDM) develop? What influences where and when perceptions germinate and become pervasive in the acceptance of the self-management of IDDM? Why is there not more encouragement to promote self-management with consideration for integrating the diabetic person's experiences and creative ideas? Has the medical community created dysfunctional dependency on their mastery of medical knowledge as the most essential factor in the self-management of diabetes? Should modern people with diabetes, having more access via technology, have the right to make decisions about their treatment? Is it time for a new paradigmatic movement, based on the activity of baby boomers who want to be able to control their lives as much as possible, independent of the old model (Bodenheimer, Lorig, Holman & Grumbach, 2010People with chronic illnesses, such as diabetes mellitus, experience management problems in their first year. There is the tedium of detail to master, and personal responsibility for well being is realized (Polonsky, 1999). Stress, burnout, and problems involving managing and living with IDDM are mentioned only briefly in the information given to diabetes mellitus patients.

Exhaustion of physical, mental, and emotional strength impairs the motivation to self-manage this chronic illness. Stress often results from the continuing challenges required to live successfully with the disorder (Sperry, 2009). Is it time for a new paradigm (Bodenheimer et al., 2010)? The literature is rich with accounts of diabetics who are mastering self-management using a new team approach. The acceleration of awareness of what diabetes is and how to control it is changing and requires a new doctor-patient paradigm. The 21st century is bringing about a renaissance in diabetic care.

Knowledgeable diabetics, eager to meet the challenges, need a new type of relationship with their healthcare providers. Bodenheimer, Lorig, Holman, and Grumbach, (2010) labeled it the patient-professional partnership. It involves collaboration and self-management education. It is important to understand this new self-management education is not a one-way system of compliance and adherence guilt trip for diabetics, but one that inspires self-efficacy and creates a desire to master individual self-capabilities to the fullest.

The intention is to understand that people with diabetes deserve to live the best possible life they are able to with a quality that exceeds the guilt laden, tedious burnout models of the past (Bodenheimer et al., 2010). The discovery of insulin was 87 years ago. Twenty-first century diabetics are yearning to be independent, not dependent on the wrinkled brow of a physician, and motivated to reach new levels of accomplishment with joy in their lives. With the large number of newly diagnosed cases of diabetes in the US today, it is an inescapable fact that the medical community is outnumbered and needs new models to meet the needs of patients. In reality, diabetics are in control, whether the doctors admit it or not.

A person with diabetes cannot not manage diabetes and live. When the diabetic goes home from the office of their health care provider, they can, and do, veto the recommendations of health professionals (Bodenheimer et al., 2010). To create eustress, diabetics must live very organized lives and maintain metabolic balance. The normalization of blood sugar positively benefits physical and mental health, reducing long-term complications and end-stage co-morbidities (Bernstein, 2007).

Distress, resulting from the tedium of managing daily blood tests, food measurement, insulin calculation, and visits to health practitioners, often results in unrelieved stress (Hirsch, 2006). The focus of this research will examine self-management in people with DM in order to provide practical and useful answers to fundamental questions in search of pragmatic and actionable knowledge, leading to successful self-management of diabetes (Guthrie & Guthrie, 2008).

Normalization of blood glucose for diabetic people is achievable by self-management (Guthrie & Guthrie, 2008). History of Diabetes Mellitus and Self-Management Sweet urine disease, later to be labeled in Latin diabetes mellitus, is described in the 110 page Ebers Papyrus scroll of 1500 BC, the writings of Celsus (30 BC–50 AD), and Chinese literature dating from 200-600 AD (Davidson, 2000). It is a metabolic disease of unknown origin, altering the endocrine hormone (insulin) secreted from the pancreas, resulting in a reduced or total inability to metabolize carbohydrates (Guthrie, & Guthrie, 2008). Paul Langerhans was the first person known to investigate the cellular systems of the pancreas.

His work in 1869 lead to the later discovery, at John Hopkins University, of islet cells in the pancreas as a secretion source for insulin in 1901 (Davidson, 2000). The internal secretion of insulin was later confirmed when it was extracted and purified from dogs in 1921 by Frederick Banting and Charley Best (Bliss, 1982). J. B. Collip discovered a formula for extracting insulin from dogs that was successful in treating Leonard Thomson, a 14-year-old, on January 16, 1922. On August 6, 1922, the Connaught and Lily Company shipped the first purified insulin in the world, leading to the successful treatment of diabetes mellitus (Bliss, 1982; Davidson, 2000). The discovery of insulin was not a cure for diabetes.

Elizabeth Hughes, the 14-year-old daughter of Secretary of State Charles Evans Hughes, was treated with insulin beginning in 1922. She later married, had children, and lived until 1981 (Bliss, 1982). It is significant to note that she required daily insulin injections for 58 years in order to live with insulin. She took approximately 43,000 injections of insulin in her lifetime (Hirsch, 2007). Diabetes Mellitus is the only major disease that is self-managed.

Elizabeth's 43,000 injections were based on her ability to follow a diabetic diet, exercise, self-test blood sugar levels, calculate the amount of necessary insulin required to normalize blood glucose, and self-inject once (or several times) daily (Hirsch, 2007). The 58 years that Elizabeth Hughes lived with IDDM was certainly dependent on the discovery of insulin by Banting, Best, and Collip. However, neither these researchers nor other health care practitioners administered the 43, 000 injections she received. Elizabeth self-injected the insulin approximately 43,000 times over a period of 58 years.

It is important to understand that IDDM is a chronic disease, requiring proactive awareness of three major tasks: self-management, role-management, and emotional management (Lorig & Holman, 2003). Since the discovery of insulin, at least one person has survived for over 80 years. James Quander was born on April 19, 1918. Quander, diagnosed with DM just before his sixth birthday in 1924, received the new insulin therapy at Freedman's hospital in Washington, D. C. He lived a full life, having married and had children, until his death on October 9, 2004. Despite the gains made by the discovery and use of insulin, diabetes remains the sixth leading cause of death in the United States, based on death certificates through 2005.

Complications of diabetes, however, are not always listed as the cause of death if other co-morbidities are involved. In 2005 there were 233,619 deaths reported as a result of diabetes (Guthrie & Guthrie, 2008). Morbidity from diabetes mellitus (DM) indicates coronary and cerebral artery disease, retinopathy, neuropathy, and nephropathy as major contributors to long-term health problems. DM is the leading cause of blindness, kidney disease, and lower extremity amputation (Guthrie & Guthrie, 2008).

This American tragedy questions the lack of involvement by the US government and third party payers to cover costs for education and ongoing monitoring costs and home management supplies (Guthrie & Guthrie, 2008). In 1925, Frederick Banting, the winner of the 1923 Nobel Prize for the discovery of insulin, stated that insulin was a treatment not a cure (Bliss, 1982). Self-management varies with age and ability. In infancy and for a toddler, self-management relies on the observation of a care-giver to monitor blood glucose, control diet, and administer insulin. Children as young as six have begun to inject themselves and master the technique of blood glucose testing under supervision.

An insulin injection error, too large a dose, can be fatal. Most people with DM wear identification bracelets, necklaces, or other identification and are aware of the need to treat hypoglycemic reactions with orange juice or dextrose tablets (Hirsch, 2006In working with chronically ill and handicapped children, Thomas L. Creer and Walter P. Christian (1976) considered the self-control of behavior proposal made by Goldiamond (1965). Motivation to take action as a skill toward one's personal health is a capability according to Bandura (1986).

Thomas Creer (1997), working with children with chronic illnesses, first used the term self-management based on Albert Bandura's publications about self-efficacy. It is easier on the emotions to handle diabetes when it is not acting-up, compared to making cognitive decisions when diabetes is not controlled. Uncontrolled, the subsequent hypoglycemic or hyperglycemic reaction produces symptomatology that is frightening or causes somnolence (Patterson, 2001). The work of self-management for IDDM involves being aware of when insulin begins to work.

There is fast-acting insulin such as Humalog, in comparison to longer acting insulin such as Lantus or Detemir; so serious attention must be paid to the quantity and mixture of insulin being used. The role of the person with diabetes is to self-test blood glucose levels and calculate an appropriate insulin dosage based on the glucose level and the quantity of food consumed. The diabetic with positive self-efficacy and an understanding that management decisions are important for future health and feelings will act.

Those experiencing defeat from the symptoms of the illness, from mismanagement, or who have not received adequate education about how to carry out the required tasks will suffer health-related co-morbidity, work loss, non-productivity, relationship problems, and financial issues (Creer & Holroyd, 2006). In a review of the literature, the self-management of diabetes offers objective viewpoints that may be plotted on a continuum with radical, perfect compliance on one side, American Diabetes Association (ADA) recommendations in the middle, and gradient levels of control (ADA, 2007; Bernstein, 2007). R. K. Bernstein (2007) maintains his personal blood glucose averages at 40%

lower than the ADA's guidelines. His office visit per patient is 3 days.

As a former engineer, Bernstein went to medical school and became an MD in order to learn how to improve management of diabetes. As a current medical practitioner, he receives clients at an office attached to his home in New York.

He maintains that his patients are happy with the health improvement and results they achieve following his educational program for managing IDDM (Bernstein, 2007). History of Self-Efficacy Models and Chronic Illness This literature review focuses on the challenge reality imposes on people newly diagnosed with IDDM and their perceptions of their ability to shape their future. People are not mere observers of life but necessarily maintain a pro-social role of fulfilling their aspirations. A diagnosis of IDDM does not change the aspirations of the person with a chronic illness, but it does require the acquisition of new skills and the strengthening of existing skills (Bandura, 1997). This section will explore the influence people have on the nature of diabetes.

For example, people cannot tell their pancreas or endocrine system what to do, but they can make decisions that provide for maximum or minimum qualities of health by utilizing personal capabilities to implement the tasks required to manage diabetes (Bandura, 1997). The literature supports indicators of self-efficacy that the diabetic person's selection of information and attention to personal capabilities is distinctive in the maintenances of a psychological quality of life. The person with DM continually adjusts and improves or avoids choices, positively or negatively, altering the physiological and spiritual quality of life.

Albert Bandura (1997) stated that people construct a belief system of self-efficacy built on four main sources of information: 1. Enactive mastery experiences. 2. Vicarious experiences. 3. Verbal persuasion and allied types of social influence. 4. Physiological and affective states. An efficacy information source provides information to a person, enabling him or her to judge or perceive personal capabilities. The means of reception and transmission of information is not essential. The efficacy information is useful only if it became instructive (Bandura, 1997).

According to Bandura, the key to efficacy information becoming instructive relies on cognitive processing and reflective thought. The process of integrating efficacy information sources into a construction of beliefs useful for the process of self-management of diabetes evaluates the trigger governing the choices, heuristics and translation of new information into personal self-appraisal abilities that become catalytic systems advancing self-efficacy and confidence to live with diabetes (Bandura, 1997). Training diabetic people to adopt a growth mind-set about mastery capabilities has a catalytic effect. It increases motivational adjustments to feel better and attain improved qualities-of-life-style experiences.

No longer are people with DM resigned to facing early death and amputations unless they are fixated on their inadequacy to solve problems and create action plans. They can begin to move in small steps toward greater freedom and independence with a once fatal, crippling disease. As a person with a chronic illness such as diabetes learns how to manage the disease with the appropriate tools, he or she becomes a health care provider with an expertise in self-management of diabetes.

Low self-efficacy, on the other hand, is characterized by being uncertain that the goal can be accomplished. By believing that one can accomplish a particular goal, the goal seeker increases the likelihood of successful behavior modeling and the likelihood that he or she will persist until the goal is achieved (Bandura, 1997). An outgrowth of Bandura's social learning theory; self-efficacy is achieved through positive past experiences, reinforcement from the environment, and encouragement from mentors. Another important factor for success is the act of observing and modeling oneself after others who have already successfully achieved the goal.

Those who expect successful achievement of goals anticipate successful outcomes. In other words, one expects to receive the benefits of achieving the goal as a result of all the hard work necessary to achieve it. Three aspects of success in academic and other life endeavors are having the necessary knowledge and skills to achieve the goal, high self-efficacy beliefs, and high outcome expectations. High self-efficacy alone does not always meet with success. Some people may have the requisite knowledge and ability to accomplish the goal and have high self-efficacy.

As a result, they can envision the successful outcome and, consequently, achieve it. Others may have the requisite knowledge and ability to accomplish the goal, but have low self-efficacy and, therefore, are not able to achieve it. Still others may think they have the requisite knowledge and ability to accomplish the goal (when in fact this is not the case), still have high self-efficacy, but fail due to the disconnect between self-perception and reality (Bandura, 1997Self-efficacy theory is reminiscent of Norman Vincent Peale's (1996) power of positive thinking.

What makes the two different is that Bandura has identified self-efficacy as a cognitive mechanism underlying all forms of psychotherapy. Therefore, self-efficacy theory could easily be placed within the learning paradigm of humanism in addition to constructivism. An outgrowth of social learning theory and of what Albert Bandura (1997) now calls social cognitive theory, self-regulated learning, as espoused by Dale Schunk and Barry Zimmerman (2001), is an essential ingredient of problem solving that is closely related to self-efficacy.

Self-regulated learners are self-motivated, self-aware, proactive learners who view the activity of learning as something they do for themselves versus something that is done to or for them. Three phases of self-regulated learning are forethought, performance, and self-reflection.

The cognitive processes involved in these three phases are: 1. Forethought: goal-setting, high self-efficacy, and strategic planning; 2. Performance: attention focusing, self-instruction, and self-monitoring; 3. Self-reflection: self-evaluation, attributions, and adaptivity (Bandura, 1997). Poor self-regulated learners have nonspecific goals, low self-efficacy, low interest in tasks leading up to goals, lack of focus, and inability to self-monitor progress. Strong self-regulated learners have specific goals, high self-efficacy, a high interest in task completion, focus, and the ability to self-monitor progress toward the goals of self-regulation (cognitivism) (Bandura, 1997). Within Alan Schoenfeld's (1992) model of mathematical problem solving, an important element to successful mathematics learning is the process of self-regulation. Self-regulation is the ability of the learner to self-monitor his or her own cognitive processes.

A technique to achieve self-regulation is the think aloud protocol, in which participants engaged in a problem-solving activity by talking out loud to share what they are thinking. A finding of the think aloud protocol was that the entire process was an exercise in mathematical metacognition, in which the participants were able to become cognizant of, supervise, and change their own cognitive processes in order to be better problem solvers and more productive at reaching their task goals (Schoenfeld, 1992).

Being able to assess personal status and progress, make adjustments to strategy, and adjust actions and procedures to meet task goals while the task is in process is essential to the self-regulation process (Davidson, 2000). A strong desire to prevent an early death by taking care of the body with 21st century self-management guidelines also reduces costs for the diabetic and the health care industry. In addition, it allows the diabetic to be more productive and contribute to society in many creative ways not thought possible just a few decades ago (Bodenheimer et al., 2010). It is no longer necessary to allow the disease to master the person.

IDDM can be successfully managed using a body of knowledge that supports well-being. Competence and security are possible in the 21st century. It is no longer necessary to accept the attitude of powerlessness and defeat.

This is a battle that can be won and there are multitudes enjoying life today because of this new paradigm of taking care of self and working in an equal collaboration with a health care provider. Self-management of diabetes (SMDM) was difficult for the first generation of surviving IDDM patients because blood and urine testing results were difficult to obtain.

The first quantitative results of a decrease in morbidities related to diabetes was reported in 1969, after the advent of a 24-hour telephone answering service provided by a health care team made up of several health care disciplines. By 1972, hospitalizations related to diabetes dropped to the same level as non-related diabetes health issues (Davidson, 2000). In 1974, podiatrists were added to the team and a 50% drop in amputations was reported. The leader in providing health care for diabetes was Grady Health System (GHS), one of the largest public hospitals in the US in Atlanta.

The GHS leadership and diabetic education program saved the American Hospital Association millions of dollars and was named the recipient of the first "National Patient Education Leader's Award for Outstanding Achievement in Patient Education Services to a Specific Target Population" in 1972. In 1997, GHS was awarded the "Quality Improvement Award by the National Association of Public Health Hospitals and Health Systems" (Davidson, 2000).

These awards and achievements however, did not reflect those Americans without healthcare or access to healthcare. The first two generations of diabetics after the discovery of insulin in 1923 suffered from morbidities related to diabetes and only a small percentage survived an early death related to diabetes. People who were diagnosed in the 1940s with IDDM are difficult to find; they have died. Diabetes is big business linking with powerful economic, social, and political forces without a clue to treatments and cures. Billions of dollars are made from selling products to diabetic clients. A treatment costs a lot of money and time for research resulting in positive changes. Until there is a cure, there is no product to market, nothing to sell.

However, a great deal of money is being made on maintaining people with diabetes: insulin, syringes, testing products, etc. The American Diabetes Association and the National Institute of Health are, in effect, stakeholders in diabetes. It is the opinion of this researcher, in agreement with Bernstein (2007) and Polonsky (2004), that if you were to eliminate diabetes, you would eliminate their careers. Empowerment gives diabetics hope and it gives them a tool for achieving problem solving skills and reducing distress by quickly trouble shooting day-to-day management of the disease. Richard Bernstein, MD, a sixty-five year survivor of diabetes, educates diabetics to emulate his success.

At age 75 he does not have diabetic complications and still maintains his practice in New York (Polonsky, 2004). At diabetes conferences, healthcare professionals are provided with information about more accurate and simpler blood glucose monitors and insulin delivery systems. The scientists providing progress reports for curing diabetes, and scientific advances are not present, however. Non-diabetics believe DM is a successfully manageable condition.

Many people believe that diabetics will live a full and normal life if they follow a correct diabetic regimen. The invention, production, and distribution by health care management insurance companies, diabetes educators, and research laboratories made blood glucose monitor available to physicians only in 1969. The monitor could report the blood glucose level of any person in 1 minute using a single drop of blood (Bernstein, 2007). The monitors cost $650 each and were sold to physicians only; none were available to people with diabetes for in-home use. While this was a great milestone, patients could get their blood glucose results only during regular scheduled visits or hospitalization.

Diabetics married to a physician, or who were physicians themselves, could order the monitor and sample their blood glucose multiple times a day. This led to the realization that in order to properly control blood glucose, information was needed: the blood glucose level. Using this information, diabetics could then adjust their insulin dosage and bring their blood glucose levels down to normal levels. However, in reality, proper control of blood glucose levels was not going to be attained simply by monitoring it.

Control required a strong desire to cope with the disease, the self-efficacy to believe in personal capacities, and money (Bernstein, 2007Good management and control of diabetes is helpful to maintain the family, especially for male and female heads of households. When diabetics experience poor control, their management skills, problem resolution capacities, family planning, social skills, and family influence diminishes.

Diabetes affects the cognitive abilities of the brain when poorly managed, and is difficult to regain acuity without good diet, exercise, and pharmaceutical management

(Puavilai & Stuifbergen, 2000). Glycemic control and quality of life, quality of family life, and quality of marital life are correlated with the level of blood glucose control in diabetic people. Diabetes is a major stressor for the diabetic, as well as for others in the family. The ability of the diabetic to manage his or her disease is essential to the quality of social relationships. When blood glucose levels have not been managed and have gotten too high for long periods of time, cognition is affected and psychological acceptance of the mental state becomes set.

Also, diabetics who over-compensate for high blood sugars and are constantly on a daily roller coaster of high and low blood sugar levels have cause for alarm. Exaggerated mental and emotional states often lead to anger, repressed emotions, and other social problems (Fisher, 2006; Trief, Himes, Orendorff, & Weinstock, 2001). When diabetics are able to manage their disease, they are able to reward themselves with self-esteem and self-efficacy that are not available to people who disregard the disease and their personal role in diabetic management. Good management results in an independence that is not available to the diabetic who relies on a spouse or others to make decisions about his or her diabetes.

While small children cannot be expected to have full control of their condition, it is essential to provide diabetic education so that, as the child matures, he or she is able to take over and control his or her own diabetes, eventually. Enabling dependence would be unhealthy for both the child and the parent.

The employability of the diabetic is also influenced by his or her ability for self-care, and thus contributes to independence and positive self-esteem, further enhancing their health. Diabetes is a disease that requires a subjective understanding of the disease, as well as education, diet, exercise, medication, and the ability to self-regulate personal behavior. Participants who have lived with diabetes for years without complications and co-morbidities were chosen for this study. Lilly pharmaceuticals and the Joslin Diabetes Center have established life awards for people who have survived lengthy periods using insulin. The "LillyforLife" program, started in 1974, currently gives awards to people who have achieved 25, 50, and 75 years as a type 1 diabetic (IDDM) (Polonsky, 2007).

One person lived with type 1 diabetes for 82 years; sixteen people for 75 years, 2200 people have lived from 25 to 50 years with the disease (Polonsky, 2007). The secret is strict control, a secret uttered by all of these survivors. However, how they did it is not widely understood because there is a paucity of literature reporting their success (Colberg & Edelman, 2007). After diagnosis of type 1 insulin-dependent diabetes mellitus (IDDM) in 1971, the author applied to the Aston Center, at the University of Texas Medical Center in Dallas, Texas, to be an experimental client of Dr. Phillip Raskin, one of the leading diabetologists in the United States.

The author participated in a double blind alductase reduction study in 1991, reported by Hanada, Kitoh, and Raskin. After one year, it was determined that there was no relation between glycemic control and either an increase in aldose reductase inhibitors or increased erythrocyte aldose reductase activity in type 1 diabetic patients (Hanada, Kitoh, & Raskin, 1991). The author also participated in genetic testing in 1999 at Neurological Associates, Baylor University Hospital, and

Richardson, Texas in 1999. The author then took part in an experiment involving Medtronic's insulin pump by other local researchers in Dallas, Texas.

It was during this period, after the 1993 DCCT trials, that Dr. R. K. Bernstein, Dr. Robert Atkins, and others began to challenge the high carbohydrate diets purported to be healthy by the American Diabetes Association (Atkins, Vernon, & Eberstein, 2004; Bernstein 2008). Dr. Bernstein went on to develop research and consulted with diabetics by phone all across the United States. He has had type 1 diabetes for 66 years and still manages the clinic in his seventies.

His diet has worked for many people and is gaining popularity with people seeking longer, better quality lives as well as a reversal of complications. Therefore, this author's theoretical orientation is in line with Dr. Bernstein as a successful 40-year survivor of DM. The main characteristic of the culturally skilled practitioner is to motivate the client to adapt this positive low carbohydrate diet. Some of the motivational techniques need to be adjusted to fit various cultures, however. Diabetes appears in all countries of the world.

It has been demonstrated that prosperity and stress are factors in newly diagnosed cases of DM, and that the human body can benefit from low carbohydrate diets (Atkins et al., 2004; Bernstein, 2008; Davidson, 2000). The purpose of this project is to integrate the psychological benefits of maintaining diabetic control using a low-carbohydrate high protein diet, integrated with motivational psychotherapy models to encourage euglycemia.

According to the literature, it appears that an intervention design, focusing on motivational interviewing (MI) has the potential for a significant reduction of the annual death rate of diabetics and accompanying comorbidities resulting from non-compliant diabetics (Atkins et al., 2004; Bernstein, 2003, 2007; Resnicow et al., 2002; Smith, Heckemeyer, Kratt, & Mason, 1997). Research supports the benefits of teaching self-management of DM using a high protein, low carbohydrate diet. Careful diet appears to be the most effective intervention leading to a better quality of life and a reduction in the death rate resulting from uncontrolled diabetes. Diabetes is an incurable, chronic disease needing management for a lifetime. An acute illness disrupts psychological and physiological health of individuals for a short time, and there are many good models for dealing with acute illnesses.

Diabetes is lifelong psychological and physiological disruption that causes behavioral complications with menses, the common cold, flu, altitude, heat, cold, stress and many other factors. There are times when people with DM need emergency attention because of acute conditions, which complicate the understanding of diabetes further for the client and medical science. It is important that scientists research a cure, but a cure may not benefit people who already have diabetes.

The models of self-management need to be dual track research designs that also provide guidance in living with diabetes (Arkowitz et al., 2008; Groeneveld, Petri, Hermans, & Springer, 1998; O'Neill et al., 2003; Snyder & Hirsch, 2008). Self-Management Behavioral Strategies to Maintain Diabetic The concept of best practices for treating diabetes does not exist in one cohesive document that the non-medical population can understand. Since the discovery of insulin in 1923, suggestions using quantitative data have emerged. Diabetic people do not live quantitative lives, but have qualitative experiences that are unique to their personalities.

The American Association of Diabetic Educators (AADE) publishes an 800-page reference manual and conducts "Core concept" seminars. However, not many can attend the seminars and most people, therefore, do not get the information. According to Dr. Richard Jackson (as cited in Tenderich, 2008) from the Joslin Diabetes Center, best practices are a consensus of ideas rather than a protocol for physiological and psychological treatment. Jackson reported that newly diagnosed diabetics receive treatment based on the preference of the hospital (Tenderich, 2008). Diabetes is an illness that requires ongoing personal work by the diabetic.

DM is not a disease that permits physical or psychological well-being unless the client is proactive in learning behaviors for coping and managing this incurable disease. In order to lessen the intensity and destructive nature of DM, diabetics must be aware of how out-of-range blood sugar levels negatively affect every cell in the human body. A compromise in the health of the brain directly affects the usefulness of the mind. It produces changes in behavior and personality, and affects the quality of personal, social, and family relationships.

The destruction of health also affects the diabetic's ability to work and produce an income (Munhall, 2001). The American Diabetes Association (ADA) and the European Association for the Study of Diabetes (EASD) advocate adding additional oral medications in combination with insulin and amylin to aid in controlling type one (IDDM) diabetes. These two large, influential associations are teaching the management of diabetes from a medical supply-side. As discussed earlier in this document, there is a long historical background of the pathophysiology of diabetes.

From 1500 BC, as translated from Egyptian Ebers Papyrus, the literature describes diabetes occurring because of eating or not eating foods. In 1921, Banting and Best discovered insulin as a treatment intervention for diabetes. They, too, advocated a low carbohydrate diet before and after their discovery. This approach remained as the modal treatment until the late 1940s. The ADA and the EASD did not integrate the DCCT trials of 1993 adequately to achieve euglycemia as the leading outcome for the majority of diabetics. ADA publishes levels of control information which is made available to the American Medical Association and the American Psychological Association.

The ADA reports that glycemic control of 7% is acceptable for self-management goals, ignoring the benefits of working to achieve long term levels of 4.5% (Accurso et al., 2008; Atkins, 2004; Bernstein, 2004, 2007; Powers, 1996; Wolpert & Anderson, 2001). Diabetes Education There are approximately 15,000 certified diabetic educators (CDE) in the United States, for over 21,000,000 people suffering with the disease. Approximately 75% of diabetics receive diabetes education in various qualities, in formats ranging from a professional educator to a friend who has diabetes.

Diabetics usually do not search for diabetes education when they must pay for it out of pocket (Powers, 1996). A national survey indicates that only 35% receive education about the self-management of diabetes through a class or special program. Diabetics using insulin (IDDM) received 10% more educational opportunities than non-insulin diabetics did (NIDDM). Friends of diabetics are providing for approximately 14% of diabetic education to fellow diabetics. The challenge to the nation is to discover a method of motivation that delivers higher results of compliance.

A large number of diabetics who receive diabetic education have difficulty understanding the seriousness of the disease. They often listen to stories from others whose family member died from diabetes, creating anxiety, depression, and ambivalence for future decisions by the diabetic. Many ignore more structured education or cannot motivate themselves to adhere to a strict regimen resulting in better health until complications develop.

There is still hope when complications begin, but the sensitivity to change is a challenge for many (Powers, 1996). Diabetic education is more useful if it empowers and awakens diabetics to practice self-management that affects their health by enabling them to maintain healthy diabetic control. Providing education without considering the enormous psychological challenge facing the diabetic is not useful. Healthy diabetic control is the ability to maintain glycosylated hemoglobin as close to 4.5% as possible. Consistent quarterly blood tests that are near 4.5% result in fewer or no complications from diabetes (Atkins, 2004; Bernstein, 2008).

Because there are obstacles that prevent diabetics receiving empowering, internal locus of control training, the most productive models remaining are evaluated: the Atkins Model, the Bernstein Model, and the American Diabetes Association Model. Dr. R. G. Atkins' (Atkins et al., 2004) research sought to link obesity and type 1 diabetes. Type 1 diabetes advances through five stages of pre-diabetic progression: weight gain, insulin resistance, and pancreatic instability, elevations of blood sugar or impaired glucose tolerance, and type 1 diabetes. Type I diabetes can occur at birth or later without pre-diabetic progression. Dr. Atkins' research is against the mainstream medical system in the United States such as the American Diabetes Association (ADA).

The ADA advocates eating a diet of carbohydrates that encourage the development of diabetes. Dr. Atkins' research and his use of a blood sugar control program seeks to advise all people and create awareness of pre-diabetic conditions in order to make dietary changes and reverse the course of the disease or control its course through self-management.

Research indicates that normal control is achievable by avoiding carbohydrates, which is at the core of diabetes, the inability to metabolize diabetes (Atkins, 2004). The best way to halt the prevalent increases in obesity and diabetes is to radically change the way we eat and live. Carbohydrates produce a pleasurable feeling in our bodies, from the stomach to the brain, but seeking psychological relief from stress by consuming carbohydrates is unhealthy. Choosing to eat what manufacturers seek to sell to the public is to choose without thinking about the health costs. Change is possible through education and motivation. Setting healthy goals that save lives from diabetes are worth it (Atkins, 2004). Dr. R. K. Bernstein (1992, 1998, 2005, and 2007) is a physician who has diabetes and has successfully managed it for more than sixty years.

His personal experiences, together with his medical education, led to the founding of a diabetes clinic in New York for the treatment of diabetes and for diabetes education. Bernstein's research supports the link between obesity and diabetes, and seeks the prevention of pre-diabetic symptoms leading to full-blown diabetes. His methods go against the mainstream establishment's methodology for the prevention and treatment of diabetes. Dr. Bernstein's (2007) 519-page book provides diabetes education for diabetics.

It is intended to permit diabetics to experience normal or near normal blood sugar levels by adopting a healthy diet, exercise, the correct utilization of medication, and frequent evaluations of glycosylated hemoglobin (Bernstein, 2007The Diabetes Control and Complications Trial (DCCT), conducted by the National Institute of Diabetes, Digestive, and Kidney Diseases (NIDDK) from 1983 to 1993, indicated for the first time in the history of diabetes the benefits of improving diabetic control (NIH, 2008). The results were dramatic. The weakness of the DCCT study was to emphasize the high cost involved in maintaining better glycemic control.

In reality, the high costs are higher by not managing diabetes. It is not expensive to manage diabetes. Effort and commitment are the only requirements. Another weakness of the DCCT trials is too little emphasis on the glycemic reduction possible to achieve. Many people with diabetes have reversed diabetes and many have achieved normal levels of blood glucose control (Bernstein, 2007). Another major weakness of this study was the recommendation of insulin therapy using one daily injection, which contradicted findings. The DCCT indicated that multiple injections were more effective in long-term improvement in hyperglycemia.

Manufacturer's literature reporting research concerning the efficacy of insulin indicates the proteins in the recombinant insulin do not replicate similarly in all diabetics. Bernstein (2007) advocates correction doses, which is an important concept for diabetics, to learn how to calculate for better control (Bernstein, 2007; Snyder & Hirsch, 2008). The DCCT trials also set in motion a schema for diabetics to control their diabetes. Control was already an important part of the diabetic regimen, but the trials triggered the promotion of tight control.

Being labeled as foolish adults or wicked children, by non-diabetic physicians and diabetic educators, negatively affects those diabetics who are unable to attain tight control and causes increased resistance to DM education. Non-diabetic others are unsure of how to understand the diabetic-self concept. The stigmatizing of diabetics who do not attain near-normal control is psychologically disabling. Depression and anxiety is a product of the impact of negative labeling (Broom & Whittaker, 2004). Type I (IDDM) diabetics need to inject insulin or take a pancreatic stimulant medication in order to live.

Diabetes increases the risk of high cholesterol and high blood pressure, and reduces life expectancy. Diabetes education that increases awareness of self-management techniques increases the potential for a diabetic to live a longer, more active and productive life (Atkins, 2004; Bernstein 2005, 2007; Munhall 2001). In addition to insulin or oral medications for diabetes, other drugs may be useful to reduce complications from diabetes. Blood pressure control, keeping blood pressure in normal ranges, can further reduce complications by as much as 40%.

Blood lipid control can reduce cardio-vascular complications as much as 50%. Laser detection equipment for the eyes and feet can prevent retinal damage and detect other neural damage (Driesen, Cox, Gonder-Frederick, & Clarke, 1995; Foreyt & Poston, 1999). The DCCT started in 1983 as a ten-year study to measure the effects of improved blood sugar levels. One of the complications of diabetes is retinopathy. The researchers were seeking to provide a method to reduce retinopathy 33%, but instead found a 75% reduction. Kidney disease was reduced 50%, nerve damage reduced 60%, and cardiovascular disease was reduced 35%.

The researchers followed a cohort of 1,441 patients for 6.5 years, after educating the clients about self-management. Outstanding results occurred among some clients, who reduced their blood sugars to normal. In addition, those who improved their blood sugars for the entire research period decreased their experience of diabetic symptoms (Diabetes Control and Complications Trial Research Group [DCCTRG], 1993). The DCCT is historically one of the most beneficial studies since the invention of insulin and the blood glucose-monitoring meter.

The published results indicate diabetics can achieve better control and experience less fear from long-term complications. The weakness of the study was it was not aggressive enough. Researchers did determine the best possible regimens with the results they collected. However, diabetics can achieve better health benefits because of the research. Some have improved by self-management, with little guidance from healthcare managers. Physicians were reluctant to be too aggressive because of the risk of hypoglycemia. Those who were too aggressive experienced hypoglycemia, but there were no fatalities.

It was difficult to find a balance with the information collected (Atkins, 2004; Bernstein, 2007; DCCTRG, 1993; Volek & Feinman, 2005). Understanding a healthy diet is essential in managing the wellness or illness of a person with diabetes. For diabetics, low carbohydrate diets are more important, and more effective, than low fat diets. This is contrary to the established teachings of the American Diabetes Association and other groups. Best practices for self-management of DM do not exist. Complications of diabetes are completely avoidable by eating correctly and managing diabetes to keep blood sugars at normal or near normal levels.

The avoidance of dairy products, grains, fruit, and high glycemic foods contributes to better health for pre-diabetic or diabetic people (Bernstein, 2005; Mayers, 2003; Wainapel, 2000). Parents and others model diets to us as children. The diets presented by our parents result in positive or negative health outcomes. Change is possible if proper dietary education explains healthy eating choices. Media advertising, vending machines, and addictive carbohydrate foods subtly suggest unhealthy choices.

Learning to choose foods that are not a psychological suggestion through the media, vending machines, and neighborhood convenient stores is a first step. Most people do not understand the proper limits of carbohydrate consumption and the damage sugar can do to the body (Bernstein, 2005). Treating hypoglycemia with a large dose of carbohydrates is an attempt to raise blood sugar. Consuming large amounts of sugar or carbohydrates to treat a hypoglycemic attack voids hormones necessary to prevent depression because they are not available.

Additionally, when blood sugars are too low or too high, the diabetic becomes too cognitively impaired, unable to choose the most effective corrective action to balance blood sugar to a normal range. A cycle of highs and lows may result in triggering a roller-coaster episode of mood swings. Each wave may result in a furtherance of incorrect choices, perpetuating emotional problems for the diabetic (Accurso et al., 2008; Akora & MacFarlane, 2005; Wainapel, 2000). In humans, euglycemia is approximately 80-120 mg/dl. Mild hypoglycemia is 55-70 mg/dl, and low hypoglycemia is 33-55 mg/dl.

Driesen, Cox, Gonder-Frederick, & Clark (1995) reported in their research that reaction time (RT) for diabetics cognitively choosing proper corrective action for hypoglycemia varies widely. When hypoglycemia occurs, the brain is not able to store sufficient neural glucose promoting consistent cognitive functions in a stable, normal pattern. This results in cortical-slowing, affecting behavior not consistent with the normalcy of the diabetic. Thus, they are frequently labeled as drunk or sleepy. Sometimes anger, too, is a reaction of hypoglycemia.

Consequently, social problems may be common when diabetes is not controlled (Volek & Feinman, 2005The physiological complexities of diabetes on the human body are a challenge to the psychological outcomes and are variables among diabetics. Knowledge about diabetes, desire for quality of life, anxiety, and depression are powerful issues that contribute to the ability of diabetics to try to become proactive in managing their disease. Health related questionnaires can assist the non-diabetic and the diabetic in understanding what motivates their selection of food products. Making food choices from habit, without thinking, often results in food selections that contribute to health risks.

Post-diagnostic testing, to measure the quantity and quality of diabetic information benefiting the client, is an important part of the intervention design. A Delphi panel is useful in helping diabetic educators determine where to begin educating a diabetic about his or her condition. Such a panel can reinforce the importance of taking care of his or her health through diet and the result if diet is ignored: unavoidable health complications and death from the disease (Bradley, 1994). Intensive or tight control for diabetes contributes to a lifestyle free from such symptoms as tiredness, high blood sugars, or anxiety about low blood sugar levels.

Roller coaster blood sugar levels contribute to irritability, anger, anxiety, and depression. Poor control results in microvascular complications and damage from non-management. Reversing complications of diabetes is possible, by using long-term compliant treatment. However, the many factors that necessitate behavioral changes may be risky for the diabetic. Goal setting should include a biological blood sugar target.

Motivation and goal setting impart empowerment to the diabetic by teaching techniques to control blood sugars versus giving in to the disease (Wolpert & Anderson,

2001). Formerly, treatment programs sought to provide tight glycemic control and avoid hypoglycemia as well as hyperglycemia. The client's lifestyle became a burden to adopt successful strategies to predict the action of insulin and meals. Flexibility and choice were not an option. Diabetes controlled the client's life. Modern methods provide and educate the diabetic with strategies to manage diabetes in order to provide more freedom, which is psychologically liberating. Designs using insulin and other medication regimens can be part of the intervention design, matching the pattern of the diabetic's lifestyle.

This has a psychological benefit of reducing depression and anxiety (Wolpert & Anderson, 2001). The Psychology of Goal Setting and Maintaining Diabetic Control Carbohydrate addiction (CA) is a diet-related disease. An evaluation of newly diagnosed cases of IDDM and the potential of carbohydrate addiction is useful as an addiction intervention, but has increasingly been useful in multiple health issues. Self-managing carbohydrate addiction (SMCA) is an integration of behavioral change theory and psychotherapy. The key strategy of SMCA is to provide viewpoints that decrease ambivalence to change.

The intervention advocates maintaining consistent control. Diabetics are more successful when they incorporate intrinsic motivation to accept adherence to a diabetic regimen as a positive behavioral choice. SMCA assists diabetics by helping them to paint a mental picture of the positive and negative outcomes of self-managing diabetes. SMCA also advocates assisting the diabetic develop an internal locus of control.

This enables people with diabetes to take charge of their minds and, consequently, take charge of their diabetes; the result is less comorbidity, extending average lifespan, and avoiding disabilities (Arkowitz et al., 2008; Atkins, 2004; Bernstein, 2007; O'Neill et al., 2003; Smith, Heckemeyer, Kratt & Mason, 1997). Approximately 30% of diabetics are able to maintain or arouse sufficient motivation to manage blood sugar levels at a level of control between 4.5% and 7%. To continue to achieve a healthy level of care, an increasing hyper-vigilance requires learning self-management techniques to manage blood sugars with appropriate diet and exercise regimens.

Increasing interest and motivation for diabetics personally choosing educational designs increases self-management abilities to live, die, or become disabled by diabetes and bring about positive changes. SMCA evaluation results may be used in the treatment of psychological issues that weaken the self-efficacy attempts of diabetic people. SMDM integrating SMCA information may arouse a trend for diabetics to reverse their declining health (Atkins, 2004; Bernstein, 2005, 2007; Snyder & Hirsch, 2008). Providing diabetic education improves the psychological condition of the client when an integration of psychotherapy and measurement assist the client in setting goals.

This scenario avoids the physician controlling DM, and puts the responsibility on the diabetic. The willingness of the diabetic to set goals toward compliance than are in agreement with the 1993 DCCT study is essential. A support system is an important component of success, but is necessarily balanced by the larger part of care responsibility placed on the diabetic willingly (Anderson et al., 1995). Anderson et al.

(1995) reported a reduction in glycemic levels for diabetics who completed a six-session patient empowerment session.

These sessions encouraged the client's ability to make positive choices using self-management that would positively affect the quality of life and psychological well-being. Patient empowerment is a motivational method of assisting clients with health problems negatively affecting their lives. Psychosocial challenges of living with a chronic disease are difficult to manage without assistance. The attitude that diabetics bring to their life's issues affects the successful reduction of glycosylated hemoglobin (Anderson et al., 1995). Goal setting is achievable by utilizing motivation to self-regulate behavior and activities to reach and sustain the desired behavioral changes.

Diabetic control and gluconeogenesis requires control through planning and self-motivation on a long-term basis. People who believe they have the ability to self-regulate their diet, exercise, and medication are more likely to be successful in managing diabetes (Bandura, 1997). People who do not think they can control problems in their lives will have difficulty-managing diabetes. In order to handle the stress of combating the disease with a challenging treatment program, the diabetic must arouse a positive mindset.

In addition, a diabetic may have such a great sense of their ability to control diabetes that they give up when goal results are disappointing (Bandura, 1997). Effective goal setting is essential in adapting health improvement strategies. Coping strategies for self-doubt and anxiety must be a part of the initial strategy. Intervention strategies for improvement in disease results, using the medical supply-side approach, are funding the development of comorbidities by accepting glycosylated levels above normal as acceptable disease management. In effect, society is funding or medicalising detrimental health habits.

Personal responsibility for goals is a more logical approach for vitality. Setting goals and self-managing lifestyles is good medicine. Personal willpower cannot change health habits. All people must self-monitor their health, rather than depend on medical professionals to prescribe medicine to feed their poor health habits (Bandura, 1998Lifestyle habits affect human health as either impairment or vitality. When lifestyle habits utilize self-management interventions from an informed source, positive benefits are experienced. Disease prevention theories affect health, including diabetes.

When bad habits are a part of an individual's lifestyle, they have to experience the misery of changing those habits in order to experience a healthy life. Controlling positive health habits in preference to bad health habits requires a strong sense of personal ability to accomplish the task. The greater the self-efficacy a person has, the longer they will be able to control negative health habits.

After some success is experienced, people are empowered by their goals, treatment plans, and life experiences (Bandura, 1998). Setting targets for diabetic control improves health when integrated with diabetic education that includes the psychological functions of setting goals and an understanding of motivation. Glycated hemoglobin and blood glucose averages are critical in achieving healthy ranges affecting cognition, quality of life, sexuality, and mood. Top down care from care providers does not enhance improvement in diabetic self-management as much as patient centered care does. Achievable targets for blood sugar control promote rapid change by using a short-step scaffolding method.

This assists results in a shorter period when the diabetic can negotiate and seek out flexibility in lifestyle choices without hampering the desired goal (Butler, Peters, & Stott, 1995). Health care professionals may not be as helpful with this model unless the diabetic has sufficient expertise to understand the detailed information required for maintaining self-management on a day-to-day basis. Ignoring diabetes for one day is not an option for a healthy diabetic. Frequent corrections within the pattern of the insulin curve or the physiology of the person are more successful than delaying corrections until an n appointment with a physician.

It can be complex for some people to grasp (Butler, Peters, & Stott, 1995). Human beings can experience motivation by setting goals for the future. By paying attention to a target or goal, the client is able to access energy to affecting health. By focusing on the task of the goal, encouraging persistence and contributing to cognition by creating strategies to improve health is essential. Psychological research indicates that when people are free to set their personal goals, a greater commitment helps them achieve success in self-management. When a task is performed, significant cognitive attention is needed to affect the outcome of the task.

Otherwise, by not deciding what are important, humans revert to relying on the arousal system (Williams, Rodin, Ryan, Grolnick, & Deci, 1998). There is a positive, linear function when the hardest goals are causal in the level of difficulty requiring the most effort from the client to achieve the target goals. When asked to do their best, clients could not function because of the lack of a reference point. Therefore, if the diabetic selects a target, they are more likely to hit it than not. Without a target, you essentially hit nothing significant except poor control.

Approaching the management of diabetes from a psychological viewpoint, most caregivers agree that motivation is critical to self-management. Success in avoiding comorbidities and complications related to diabetes, including quality of life, requires careful planning.

Diabetics who are more self-efficacious in goal setting are more successful in maintaining control of diabetes and are empowered to continue and sustain self-care and self-management with more positive health outcomes and fewer co-morbid complications in long-term diabetes (Williams et al., 1998). Self-Management Psychology of Diabetic Identity and Diabetic Control The target population for this project is diabetics who are managing their disease with guidelines proposed by non-diabetics. Diabetic advisement is commonly a referral of recommendations from the American Diabetes Association. The preblockedion of ADA guidelines are given with no regard to comparison with other successful programs that have lower rates of comorbidities and a higher success rate of blood sugar control (Totty, 2008). The ADA does not take into consideration the carbohydrates available to early humans.

Their recommendation of 130 grams of carbohydrates is impossible to control with insulin and avoid obesity (Bernstein, 2007). Diabetes results in changes to the body that promotes intuitive introspection. These changes in body awareness make educational awareness more successful, also. The goal of this project is to create awareness among diabetics. They can have a higher quality of life, live healthier, and longer than predicted by the ADA. Diabetics in metropolitan environments have more access to diabetic education.

Therefore, one suggestion would be to mail compact discs with diabetic educational materials from diabetic supply companies and pharmacies; replicate of The Diabetes Bus is another viable option for advancing the promotion of diabetes education (Tenderich, 2008; Totty, 2008). Carbohydrate restriction has been historically the main model of treating diabetes since before Hippocrates until the ADA promulgated high carbohydrate diets in the 1940's (Westman, & Vernon, 2008). The treatment of diabetes with high carbohydrate diets are resulting in malpractice lawsuits.

Research indicates that by comparison amputation, blindness, kidney disease and other comorbidities known as the metabolic syndrome are a result of high carbohydrate diets (Mayer, 2003; Wainapel, 2000). The target population includes diabetics that have been recommended high carbohydrate diets since the 1940's. From the late 1940's until the 1993, DCCCT high cholesterol was an unproven hypothesis that complications from diabetes came from high cholesterol. Current research concludes that for diabetics low carbohydrate diets decrease cardiac risk factors. The ADA opposed self-blood glucose monitoring (BGSM) for 14 years.

The ADA continues to recommend "industrial doses of insulin" Medicare will not pay for BGSM (Bernstein, 2007).

Realistic goals other than perfection are essential in success with diet, exercise, and management of diabetic medication. People that are easily disappointed because their goals are not attainable as quickly will self-destruct and not regard any positive, high quality goal setting. Personal identity as a perfectionist may lead to impulsiveness, depression, and anxiety because diabetes self-management is a life led by numbers.

One track of a health habit or lifestyle will not result in changing all the adaptations a diabetic must incorporate into their identity to be successful in self-managing their disease (Foreyt, & Poston, 1999). Diabetes presents hyperglycemia when not controlled by insulin or oral medication. Approximately 90% of diabetics are obese. High carbohydrate diets and a sedentary lifestyle contribute to this problem. In that comorbidities between diabetes and obesity exist, it is essential to understand diets adequate to achieve normalization of blood sugars. Lifestyle changes must include self-monitoring of blood glucose, exercise, and coping skills to avoid anxiety and depression. Goal setting and diabetes education are also important.

People who alter their diet and lifestyle increase their quality of life and benefit from increased cognitive behavior and skills. Tests indicate that high blood sugar levels interfere with synaptic efficiency in the brain and interfere with axon potential throughout the body (Foreyt & Poston, 1999Diabetics with a perfectionist tendency are a risk to their health. Self-efficacy is significant in the diabetic's ability to address issues and develop problem-solving skills. Barriers to goal achievement occur as illnesses other than diabetes that decrease or complicate the ability to control blood sugar levels.

Hospitalization for other health issues, not related to diabetes, can disrupt the diabetic's ability to self-manage unless previous communication with the physician and care team is in place. In order to cope with change in employment, income, relationships, and other emotional issues, diabetics need a plan to prevent giving up on previously gained successes. Reaching out for social support is significant.

Tight control can be fatal without insight to the nature of diabetes (Heisler, Piette, Spencer, Kieffer, & Vijan, 2005). Self-Management, Self-Efficacy and Intentional Control Therapy (ICT) Motivational Interviewing (MI) is increasingly successful in assisting people deal with health problems that have psychological implications when related to pathology (Franken, 2002). MI is effective in reducing ambivalence toward change, encouraging commitment, and learning how to acquire the mental energy for change. Using MI as a pretreatment strategy is the intervention of choice. Pretreatment is more effective in producing cognitive changes in behavior towards self-management. The pretreatment phase of diabetic education may enhance the ability of the diabetic to make changes.

Clients who have low motivation to make positive changes toward self-management may need additional cognitive therapy before motivational results are attainable (Arkowitz et al., 2008; Franken, 2002). The key strategy to maintaining control is to develop intrinsic motivation to adhere to a diabetic regimen.

Using MI to resolve ambivalence, to plan strategies, and arrange personal support systems and strategies for increased control of diabetes increasing glycemic control of diabetes leads to better psychological health and quality of life (Arkowitz et al., 2008). In understanding the theory of change, diabetics can invest their time and effort into a healthier life leading to increased quality of life for self, family, workplace, and society. Using ICT actions, habits, aspirations, dreams, feelings, and perceptions need focus toward a sustainable level for a lifetime instead of short-term compliances with diabetic care. The client may need an epiphany or a catastrophe in order to evoke the deep needed wisdom to change life style health habits involving eating, exercise, thinking, and addictions.

Without change, a diabetic will experience the boiling frog effect by remaining unaware of nerve damage until it is too late to do anything about their condition (Boyatzis, 2006; Munhall, 2001). Change requires an "investment of energy" in order to reach a level of sustained change. It is human nature for humans to change their minds, thinking, and habits. However, the physiology, in the case of diabetes, responds to blood glucose control based on the intake of food and medicine, combined with exercise and work. The ideal self versus reality, strengths, weaknesses, learning design, willingness, and commitment to intervention adjustments is essential for success (Boyatzis, 2006).

The perception of self-confidence and cognitive skills, including aptitude, are significant indicators towards the success of self-care. In this respect, aptitudes are more important than self-efficacy. It is essential for optimal functioning. Self-determination and the diabetic's voluntary participation in changing diet, exercise, and medication behavior are the foundation of a successful construct and goal success (Anderson et al., 1995; Boyatzis, 2006). Complying with goal setting is not easy. Difficult goals may cause the reverse of desired effects.

Interventions that provide goals to the client on paper may be out of range for the ability of the spirit of the person to comply. One technique is for the client to write vigorously about desired goals and modify the approach to what is achievable in small chunks. This helps the diabetic advance slowly, but surely, for a life term change, rather than a temporary change with a relapse. Personal and family factors associated with quality of life, especially for adolescents, may intervene.

Adolescents with diabetes, who seek to please the doctor with good blood sugar readings, are less successful than diabetics who are autonomous in their choice to self-manage and self-regulate their eating and lifestyle behaviors. This is typical in adolescents, who also experience more depression because of not being able to self-regulate, and who feel inferior to their non-diabetic peers and family members (Bernstein, 2007; Broom, & Whitaker, 2003). The significance of metabolic control needs national attention through the media, health insurance companies, physicians, diabetic educators, and advertising. Diabetes education needs to be a mandatory part of any diagnosis of diabetes.

Education in high school and college health classes would have an impact. Doctors also need training on how to provide diabetic education. Giving a client an appointment, a blood test, and a bill is not sufficient. Most physicians assume diabetic control is acceptable at rates 200 to 300% over normal limits for healthy physiological and psychological needs. Research reporting how diabetes affects the brain in longitudinal studies is scarce. A significant trend in modernity is the graduating increased diet up to 60% and 70% because of carbohydrate addiction.

It is widely known in the medical community that an excessive intake of carbohydrates results in abnormal blood sugars. A consistent bombardment to the endocrine system of humans with consumption of carbohydrates 1000% above the needs of the body weakens and destroys the body's capability to metabolize carbohydrates.

The pancreas does not have a limitless supply of insulin and amylin to facilitate the digestion of carbohydrates without anoxerient medication (Bernstein, 1992, 1998, 2007; Driesen et al., 1995; Powers, 1996). Cognitive behavioral intervention education and personal therapeutic design models are promising for helping adolescents, and adults, suffering from an inability to achieve consistent euglycemia. Euglycemia is a blood sugar range conducive to a consistent level of glucose supply to neurons. The ability to cope with anxiety and the diabetic's personal perception of his or her disease often produces unexplainable behavior, resulting in social and personal problems. The relative risk (RR) of experiencing hypoglycemia is influenced by any increase of insulin of 0.1 U/kg per bodily weight, correlating with an RR of 1.07.

Therefore CBT (cognitive behavioral therapy), combined with diabetes education about the physiological wave response of insulin, should be researched further. This combination should assist diabetics make corrective adjustments to bring down hyperglycemic readings in order to avoid a corresponding hypoglycemic reaction at the end of the response cycle of the insulin (Hains, Davies, Parton, & Silverman, Clients who are proactive in requesting diabetic education from educators familiar with cognitive behavioral therapy (CBT) indicate significant improvement of anger management also. An anger temperament is an indicator of blood sugars outside the euglycemic range of non-diabetes.

An improvement in trait anger using CBT reduces cardiovascular complications; atherosclerosis and carotid artery problems are proportionately parallel to the improvement of any improvement of anger. Behavioral research needs more funding and encouragement from diabetic drug companies. Also important are comparison studies of results based on culture, socioeconomic status, and the ability of the diabetic to be motivated. The client may need anti-depression or anti-anxiety drugs. CBT offers the opportunity for diabetics to confront denial of their treatment approach.

Myths, ambivalence to change, and personal perception of success with current self-management of diabetes are a key design factor (Golden et al., 2006; Resnicow et al., 2002). The successful programs of Atkins and Bernstein, in comparison with the American Diabetes Association and the US Department of Health and Human Services, provide statistical research for diabetics desiring a choice between more successful diabetic education models. Improve the methods that the public and private sectors fund in diabetic research.

Diabetics with other metabolic diseases require subtle planning, differing from clients with diabetes only. Other diseases affect the need for even more education (Bernstein, 2004, 2008; Powers, 1996). The research of Westman & Vernon, (2008) provided data that support intensive control. Their research indicated intensive control is not responsible for the increased risk, but rather is the method to obtain tight control.

When large amounts of carbohydrates are treated with high insulin dosages, the risk of death from hypoglycemia and cardiovascular reactions are increased (Acurso et al., 2008; Akora & McFarlane, 2005; Volek & Feinman, 2005). Since there are no established best practices for treating diabetes or educating diabetics, the disease remains one of self-management. In the 21st century, more physicians and educators are adopting the low carbohydrate regimen. However, when choices made by diabetics are left up to the illness or the diabetic self, the choice is one of life or death, disability or mobility, psychological problems or psychological health, and progress. Diabetic education is not simply handing out information to a newly diagnosed client.

An intervention using the Understanding the Model of Self-Care Decision Making (UMSCDM), is useful (Munhall, 2001). The UMSCDM integrates personal theorizing using other tools for diabetics to make good choices. People who are uncertain may be afraid to make changes on their own. This is an asymptomatic problem, because diabetics who are not succeeding with the advice of physicians often internalize their efforts as incorrect. They do not consider the experience the doctors has with DM or if diabetic education was a part of his or her degree. Some doctors merely hand out printed material, expecting the client to understand it.

That is not diabetic education (Munhall, 2001). In summary, the self-management of diabetes is best classified as a response. Three specific management-types are presented by Kelleher (1988). 1. Copers are motivated to assume as much control as possible over diet, exercise, insulin management, and injection times. The self-efficacious motivation to maintain the highest level of control as possible is present in order to work and maintain a social life, without compromising or changing their previous level of energy investment. 2. Normalisers are less disciplined but consider their approach adequate to avoid co-morbidities.

Normalisers still test their blood glucose frequently, but more for compliance rather than for micro-managing blood glucose levels. The changes they have made to life and quality of life experiences are considered satisfactory. 3. Worriers and agonisers, according to Kelleher (1988), carry a sense of being unhealthy, no matter what their investment is in diabetes self-management. They worry about having diabetes and often question their ability to manage the disease. In reality, they may be doing as well as copers and normalisers, but do not have confidence in their capacities or self-efficacy to do well.

Maclean (1991) presented the self-management of diabetes among IDDMs plotted on a continuum. She presented the levels on the continuum as: 1. Strict adherence. 2. Moderately flexible. 3. Very flexible. 4. No adherence. Maclean (1991) observed that people newly diagnosed with diabetes are most likely to micro-manage the disease in the early stages, and if they don't suffer from burnout, will continue on some level of stricter self-management practices. Some labeled their management as giving themselves permission to cheat on their diet sometimes and indulged in junk food.

They still maintained a high level of self-efficacy, which added to their confidence in living well with diabetes. Very flexible managers were those who used larger dosages of medication to comply. The no-adherence groups considered themselves obsessed with food. Some ate extra food because they were afraid of hypoglycemic reactions. They were similar to the agonisers and worriers clients described by Kelleher (1988). Some people with diabetes have a high desire to avoid short term symptoms.

Therefore, they were not looking at long-term co-morbidities, but seeking to live as pleasurable life as possible by avoiding high or low blood glucose levels. This group is straddlers, lying between Kelleher's (1988) copers and normalisers, or Maclean's (1991) moderately flexible and very flexible. Those seeking to avoid long-term consequences of diabetes consider diabetes as a serious chronic illness and require strict control, regardless of the symptoms of feeling uncomfortable with their methodology, as long as the laboratory numbers for blood glucose averages and other indicators of health were within the normal range for the general population.

Some in this group said they cheated but did not over-cheat. Physicians and researchers have classified the cause of diabetes as being genetic, viral, immune issues, because of obesity, or metabolic problems. Physicians have not appeared to consider the psychological and social support the diabetic needed in order to incorporate self-efficacy attempts to live with the illness. Qualitative research does not show up in the literature as research that physicians would consider as part of the management strategy nor provide education related to anything other than quantitative studies.

For example, if the ADA reported a blood glucose average of 6% as necessary to avoid complications, physicians would follow that advice. If the ADA changed the level to 7%, the majority of physicians would use this as a threshold. The same reasoning has been applied to hypertensions levels and other metabolic reports (Campbell et al., 2003). It has been noted that diabetic people often began their diabetic journey without considering the seriousness of the disease and reversed their attitude after living with the effects later.

Pessimism and optimism were prevalent among all diabetics, but optimism was reported higher among those who experienced more self-efficacy in other areas of their life as well as diabetes. The more experience a diabetic has with diabetic outcomes, as related to daily behavior and feelings of well-being, the more self-efficacy levels became prevalent as part of their involvement in self-management. Insights into successful management of diabetes were more evident in qualitative reporting than looking to quantitative results only.

Quantitative reports reported only numbers or levels of control without being able to relate the outcome to a self-management technique or psychological relationship to self-efficacy (Campbell et al., 2003). Conclusion The researcher concludes that the literature reports barriers to both self-management and self-efficacy that contribute to the success of self-care required for optimal glycemic control and to behavioral issues. Self-efficacy requires the belief that planning for meals, hypoglycemic attacks, how to eat out, and what emergency food to carry is used, and is not just a vague mental awareness. The person diagnosed with DM also has a level of self-efficacy that positively expresses confidence in insulin and in their physician to provide accurate advice and care.

In addition, self-assertiveness is necessary to meet the needs of the predictable and unpredictable nature of diabetes. A disagreement with one's personal physician is a positive quality in building self-efficacy and self-management skills. A measurement is non-productive if the person with diabetes is unhealthy and experiencing psychological pain. CHAPTER 3. METHODOLOGY Introduction The researcher proposes a generic-qualitative approach of inquiry.

The study's procedures consist of a qualitative evaluation of factors and characteristics important in the self-management of Type I (IDDM) diabetes. The participants will be from a non-randomized, purposive, convenience sampling of diabetics responding to a simple poster/notice on a white letter size piece of paper. The poster/notice will state that the researcher is seeking diabetic people to interview and will be displayed in endocrinologists' offices randomly selected from the Dallas, Texas metropolitan area.

The foundational method of thematic analysis is proposed to determine themes in participants' meanings following informal, face-to-face interviews, with notes made by the researcher during the interview (Braun & Clarke, 2006). The interviews will be audio-taped and transcribed, analyzed and kept in a safe deposit box or locked file box for seven years and then destroyed. The researcher proposes a generic qualitative approach. The researcher will prepare a copy of the research study, and a poster advertising the study and seek permission to display the poster/notice in the endocrinologists' offices. Ten participants will be interviewed and the data will be collected in a series of at a reserved room at a public library. The interview will be audio-taped and transcribed.

This data will be kept in a safe-deposit box or locked file box for seven years and then destroyed. Purpose of Study Restated The first purpose of this study is to identify qualitatively, utilizing a generic-qualitative method, how people with diabetes mellitus acquire health-literacy. The second purpose of this study is to determine the manner in which self-management expertise is learned. The final purpose of this study is to collect generic-qualitative information on improving the health-literacy process. Population The population of interest for this study is people with type 1 diabetes.

Diabetes is a disease that requires a subjective understanding of the disease. In addition, the patient requires education, diet, exercise, medication, and the ability to self-regulate personal behavior. The participants will self-select by responding to a notice placed in the offices of at endocrinologists' in the Dallas, Texas metropolitan area. Ten Type I (IDDM) diabetics will be selected at random from volunteers completing a self-motivated telephone call to the researcher who has read the advertised poster indicating their desire to participate.

Demographics With regard to self-selection, any adult person who has been diagnosed with type I (IDDM), regardless of race, culture, or religion, is a candidate for participation. There is no criterion for length of time for the diagnosis. The diagnosis of (type 1) diabetes may have been made recently or years before. The preferred age range for participants will be 25 to 75 years of age. Children will not be solicited or accepted into the study. Participants will be English speaking, to avoid translation difficulties. Participants must be at least 25 years of age and not more than 75 years of age.

Sampling Procedure Recruiting A convenience sampling of participants with type I (IDDM) diabetes mellitus will be used for this research. Posters will be placed in the offices of endocrinologists in the Dallas, Texas metropolitan area explaining the study and describing all ethical requirements. Included will be a consent form and an explanation that participants will receive a $25.00 gift card for completing an estimated 60 to 90 minute interview in a private room at a public library.

Convenience sampling is a technique that allows the researcher to recruit participants specifically available to the researcher (Morse & Richards, 2002). Endocrinologists specialize in treating the endocrine glands and the disease of diabetes. At least three offices will be considered for placement of the poster recruiting potential participants. Given an anticipated N of 10, three offices will provide a wide enough base and sufficient numbers of potential participants. Recruitment is the responsibility of the researcher, who will prepare and deliver a copy of the research proposal, and a poster advertising the study for consideration to several endocrinologists' offices.

The researcher will also discuss with support staff a method for poster maintenance. Upon acquiring a sufficient number of participants, data will be collected in one-on-one interviews.

After all interviews are conducted, the researcher will send copies of the taped interviews to a professional transcriptionist. The recruitment materials will include information (name, phone number, and e-mail address) for the prospective participant to use to contact the researcher Selection A screening is conducted by the researcher asking the potential participant to affirm they have been diagnosed by a medical doctor that they are a Type I (IDDM) diabetic person to insure that potential participants are: 1. A Type I (IDDM) diabetic person between 25 and 75 years of ager with type I (IDDM) diabetes. 2. Affirm that they are willing to sign a consent form protecting their confidentiality by asking them the question. 3. Affirm that they understand the researcher's presentation of the research proposal and their volunteer participation in the study by signature. Sample Size There is no upper limit on the number of potential participants who might volunteer to assist this researcher.

However, once all potential participants have been screened, as described above, only 10 names will be used to participate in one-on-one interviews with the researcher. Ten people are an adequate sample for qualitative research purposes where each participant will be interviewed in-depth. Dr. Makatura and Dr. Sarnoff have indicated fewer are acceptable.

The committee suggested it is more doable with 3 or 4 clients. Discussion The purpose of this research is to collect and report the results of an in depth qualitative study designed to understand the psychology of Type I (IDDM) diabetes self-management consistent with social cognitive theory. Thus, the generic themes will be guided by the themes of social cognitive theory.

Subjects will not be coerced or pressured to participate, either during recruitment or during the interview (NIH, 1979). The participants will be offered the opportunity to contact the researcher at any time concerning the research. The research is open and each participant may agree or not to meeting together at the conclusion of the research for questions and sharing the results of the study. Respect for persons will be ethically and professionally maintained at all times with a record of all contact, including location and means (mail, telephone, etc.), maintained for the research.

This is not to say the researcher should conduct biased shaping of the collected material, but he should provide enough clarification so others understand any new conclusions that emerge have been filtered out of the researcher's personal history with the topic of study (Kostere & Percy, 2006). In addition, the researcher should not attempt to coerce or position questions or lend interpretations to create an expected answer, but rather should provide clear, open-ended questions and listen.

If the researcher provides the participant with an interpretation of the question, that fact needs to be noted in the saved edition and included in the study (Kostere & Percy, 2006). This researcher has experience in using bracketing and epoche. The researcher conducted research for Eastfield College in Mesquite, Texas, each semester for three years to obtain information about the new student orientation designed by the researcher. In order to do this, focus groups were organized and conducted. All information was audiotaped and transcribed. Themes were analyzed and listed and presented to the Dean of Student Services (Shipman, 2005). It is the responsibility of professionals to "police their own" and provide guidelines to protect the interviewee and client from harm (Bersoff, 2003).

The interview method will be used to explore the person's experiences of living with diabetes mellitus. Methodology The researcher will interview the randomly selected type 1 diabetics. Open ended and semi-structured questions will be used during the interview. Each interview will be audiotaped, with the full knowledge and consent of the people being interviewed. The resulting audio tapes will be transcribed. All editions will be viewed and reviewed to identify nodes, themes and patterns for thematic analysis following the outline of the data collection methodology given in the MRF. Generic qualitative inquiry for the purpose of this research question was chosen in order to produce the greatest clarity about the self-management of diabetes from the perspective of the diabetic. Qualitative research uses reflections, thoughts, opinions, attitudes, and beliefs willingly shared, without the shaping influence of the researcher. Embedded themes are sought by the researcher, critically thinking about the self-report of the diabetic participant.

In discussing their individual processes of self-management, participants with DM will give voice to previously unacknowledged pieces of the story of diabetes. Therefore, the researcher is active in seeking the themes (Braun & Clarke, 2006). The researcher's rationale for this approach is based on pre-knowledge and pre-understanding of diabetic self-management. This researcher seeks to describe more fully the topic of self-management (Kostere & Percy, 2006).

The units of analysis for this study will be the individuals' thoughts, attitudes, beliefs, issues, and reflections that have shaped the self-regulatory capacity (Bandura, 1986) of the self-management of diabetes. Ethical Considerations The researcher does not anticipate any ethical concerns since interviews will be in public areas of the participants' choosing, e.g. A public library conference room. A consent form and orientation of the research will be explained. No coercion or attempt to skew the participants' freedom of expression will be used.

At the end of the dissertation procedure, the research results and a copy of the study will be available to each participant requesting a copy. Participants will be informed of the nature of the research and of their freedom to participate, withdraw, or decline the interview person that contacts you could be screened on the phone and then accepted. After a sufficient number of participants, any other individuals who call will be told that sufficient volunteers have been recruited but their name will be put on a reserve list in the event the researcher would require additional participants. The open-ended questions will be presented to the participant for preview before presentation of the consent form.

All persons will be presented with the potential harm, risks, and benefits. All persons agreeing to participate will be included in a list of potential subjects and participants will be selected randomly from that list. This avoids favoring any demographic range of participants. There will be no coercion or pressure to participate during the interview or during any attempt to recruit subjects (NIH, 1979). The participants will be offered the opportunity to contact the researcher at any time concerning the research.

The research is open and all participants may agree to meet together at the conclusion of the research for questions and sharing the results of the study. Respect for persons will be ethically and professionally maintained at all times, with a record of all contact, including location and means (e-mail, telephone, etc.) maintained for the research.

Audio tapes will be preserved in a safe-deposit box at the researcher's bank. Data Collection The data collection method using open-ended, semi-structured interview questions from IDDMs is appropriate in learning the issues, factors, and characteristics of behavioral attunement toward improving skills to self-manage diabetes (Kostere & Percy, 2006). The study of diabetes mellitus and the self-management process will proceed by using an open-ended questionnaire during a 60–90 minute audio-taped interview, one participant at a time. Ten participants will be sought. Participants will be those that self-manage IDDM. All of the interviews will be audio taped and transcribed.

All field notes will also be typed and considered for input for discourse analysis of the material (Kostere & Percy, 2006). The following questions will be asked of each person1. What are the most important lessons Type I (IDDM) diabetics have learned that have contributed to success in the self-management of diabetes mellitus? 2. What educational experiences are useful in learning about the self-management of Type I (IDDM) diabetes mellitus? Who or what is the most helpful? 3. What have other Type I (IDDM) diabetics reported that is helpful? 4. What has the medical community reported that is helpful? 5. What has the American Diabetes Association reported that is helpful? 6. What spiritual resources have been helpful? 7. What has self-study and self-education contributed? 8. What has been and is most useful to success in managing diabetes mellitus.

9. What happens when self-management of Type I (IDDM) diabetes is not working or does not bring about the expected results? 10. What goals are essential for Type I (IDDM) diabetes management? 11. What is useful in constructing a Type I (IDDM) diabetes regimen for self-management of diabetes mellitus? 12. What positive strengths are useful that have contributed to success in living with diabetes? 13. What is the most challenging thing that has happened to you as a result of being a diabetic? 14. What impact do family, friends, and peers have in diabetic self-management experience? 15. What is currently useful in improving diabetes self-management? 16. What advice is needed for diabetics experiencing diabetes? 17. Are the experiences of social stigma from being a diabetic significant and, if so, how? 18. What were the most difficult challenges in adapting to being a diabetic and managing the disease? 19. Which support system is the most effective for living with diabetes and how helpful is it? These questions, and any additional questions which might arise during the course of an interview, will permit the researcher to describe more fully the diabetics' perspective of self-management. The diabetics' reports of "their subjective opinions, attitudes, beliefs, or reflections on their experiences" of self-management will be investigated (Kostere & Percy, 2006, p. 7). Data Preparation

Data Analysis The research will be written for the purpose of contributing to the body of knowledge that others may use to research self-management of IDDM. The study does not mandate truth or certainty. The research is not intended to conclude with a list of do these things and you will live well with diabetes. The research will stimulate further research on the IDDM long-term experience. Inductive analysis will be used interpret the data avoiding pre-conceptual formation of categories. Color coding of themes will be organized into groups called nodes of analysis.

These clusters will be described and identified for patterns. These patterns will be organized into an overall matrix that is coded and diagramed with labeling identifying the factors and characteristics of each. The intention of this process is to synthesize all data from each question into a composite understanding of the experience (Kostere & Percy, 2006). The open ended interview questions will be used to enhance the credibility in the analytic process. An obvious avoidance of assumptions and minimal reliance of in vivo quotations will be utilized to over determine a pattern of information.

The goal is to thoughtfully interpret the results and explain the quality of the conceptual information (Thorne, Kirkham, & O'Flynn-Magee, 2004). The researcher's insight of participant input of data will be presented by organizing the characteristics, factors, and best practices of those interviewed.

Following this, the researcher will present a summary of the analysis of the study (Braun & Clarke, 2006). Theoretical Assumptions This researcher proposes that Albert Bandura's (1986) social cognitive theory is an explanation that translates how personal behavior, environment, and personal cognitive factors are exemplary of the nature of humans living with a chronic disease. Topical Assumptions This researcher proposes the literature from the past 90 years is indicative of the difficulties encountered when managing insulin-dependent diabetes mellitus (Banting, 1922; Galmer, 2008; Guthrie, & Guthrie, 2008; Tattersall, 2009). Methodological Assumptions Research utilizing thematic analysis provides rigor, themes, and patterns in relation to epistemological and ontological positions that are useful and flexible (Kostere & Percy, 2006).

The product is not assumed to be scientific, certain, or the last words in understanding the self-management of type I (IDDM) diabetes. Thematic analysis provides an approach to methodological data with rigor. It offers the researcher an opportunity to be explicit and clear about what the researcher is doing. Thematic analysis requires that what is attempted is in accord with the proposal.

It is a good fit for qualitative research of diabetes mellitus and self-management because the researcher may write with balance and consistency for the epistemological intent of the study (Kostere & Percy, 2006). Unexpected insights may emerge, providing an opportunity for comparison of the data with the literature review. These insights may contribute to the development of institutional policy regarding the self-management of Type I (IDDM) diabetes (Braun & Clarke, 2006; Popper, 1986). Expected Findings Physicians make diagnoses of Type I (IDDM) diabetes. The patients are then advised of the most current guidelines to treat the disease. However, the subjective opinions, beliefs, attitudes, and self-reflections come from within the mind of the diabetic.

This researcher seeks to collect these subjective expressions and thematize them, looking for information that is not a generalization. This researcher considers a quantitative approach to be a generalization and not helpful to other diabetics because it is not expressed in the language of the diabetic. The goal of this researcher is to learn about the self-management of diabetes from the perspective of the diabetic. Using thematic analysis in a generic, qualitative inquiry, the researcher will examine viewpoints, thoughts, and reflections to understand diabetes self-management.

Generic themes are not decided upon prior to the interview, but will require filtering linguistically and thematically in order to organize them into a pattern consistent with comprehension (Braun & Clarke, 2006This researcher seeks a holistic and integrated understanding of diabetics' opinions, attitudes, beliefs, and reflections about self-management of their lives and living with diabetes. After transcribing recordings of the open-ended interviews, the researcher will read and organize the material. Initial impressions will be noted, and a search for themes will follow. Themes will be extracted and coded.

A thematic map of the analysis codes, including a deblockedion of the process and rationale for each code, will be created. The themes will be refined and reviewed. Deblockedions and definitions will be derived and analyzed. The researcher will produce a report of the analysis, relating to the research question, written in a scholarly manner supported by the literature (Braun & Clarke 2006). This information will be obtained from interviews with Type I (IDDM) diabetics. The interviews will be audiotaped, transcribed, analyzed, thematized, and explained in a written narrative.

The researcher will seek data concerning the self-management of Type I (IDDM) diabetes and identify qualities of self-regulatory capabilities. In qualitative research, the researcher cannot go into the research assuming to find something;

it has to emerge from an analysis of the research after the tranblockeds are typed.

Purpose of the Study The purpose of this study is to obtain a better understanding of the personal experiences of insulin dependent diabetics (IDDM) working within a managed care health system to identify "what factors and characteristics are important in self-management of diabetes?" While this study involves self- management and learned techniques of applied self management of a chronic illness it is ultimately a study on how people with an incurable disease adapt to change when the level of personal involvement and belief is high. Of particular interest is the person living with IDDM and how they process information from health managers as people in making decisions and choices who may be limited by their ability to personally experience IDDM. This decision-making ability places the physician in a position of potential control over the client's choices for self-management and future health.

The data was collected from 11persons volunteering in a study advertised at Parkland Diabetes Clinic, Dallas, Texas. Participants were interviewed utilizing the 19 questions approved for the study regarding their self-management experience in a reserved room at Carrollton, Farmers Branch, or Dallas public libraries. This information was digitally recorded, transcribed and analyzed in an attempt to understand how these IDDM participants coped with the self-management of their illness. The participants all shared stories of self=management.

Part of the intent of this research project was to analyze the responses of persons age 35-75 that are IDDM, and compare the emergent themes with those of Albert Bandura's social learning theory Bandura concludes that ignoring the power of self-reinforcement in self regulation of health behavior is to "disavow a uniquely human capacity" (Bandura, 1974). To do otherwise conditions individuals toward possessing learning bias empowering disability. The results of this study support Bandura's results, support Kanfer (1975). Adjustment to managing a chronic illness such as IDDM requires targeting and monitoring self-monitoring and self-observation.

A deliberate commitment to "attend to one's own behavior" is mandatory not a coincidence (Kanfer, 1975). Methodology The researcher used a generic qualitative design interview focus as the research methodology. This methodology was chosen because it provided a process to capture the feelings or attitudes about a particular experience without the theoretical framework of other qualitative methods (Percy & Kostere, 2008).

Caelli, Ray, and Mill (2003) describe generic qualitative research as an approach used when the researcher is either combining a number of approaches or aiming no specific methodological perspective. Caelli et al. also describe this methodology useful when the "focus of the study is on understanding an experience or event" (p.4). The focus of this research was to obtain an understanding of the attitudes and experiences of case managers as they adapt to change in their primary role.

A generic qualitative methodology allowed the researcher the structure and ability to ask open-ended questions without assigning a philosophical perspective. The researcher used content thematic analysis utilizing an objective interpretation of meaning units as a model to condense the meaning units into a unified theme. (Graneheim & Lundman, 2003). Thematic analysis was used to ascertain, examine, and describe patterns within the data (Braun & Clarke, 1006). Data Collection Data collection consisted of several steps. The researcher first obtained permission to conduct the study from the Parkland Diabetes Medical Clinic, Dallas, TX. The Parkland Diabetes Medical Clinic, Dallas, TX, is the administrative agency that oversees the care of people with diabetes that cannot pay for their care. The researcher contacted the director, Dr.

Phillip Raskin about study participation and he supported and agreed to help and agreed to participate. After obtaining these permissions, the researcher requested Institutional Review Board (IRB) permission. Once IRB permission was granted, the researcher posted an information page about the study and waited for participants to make contact to set up a place to conduct an interview directed by the approved IRB questions. The researcher handed out informed consent forms and collected the forms from participants that agreed to research participation.

All together 10 participants with IDDM participated in the research. All participants provided the researcher with confirmation of their diagnosis of IDDM by an endocrinologist. Since this study was interested only in the fact that the participants were age 25 -75 participants shared their ages. Eleven participants were interviewed. The interviews took place in a place in a reserved library. In spite of this, the participants showed a great deal of ease and comfort. This was a public and open environment and participants were informed of the choice to withdraw from participation. There were none that did.

The interviews took place over a span of four months. Appointments were scheduled as soon as possible as convenient to the participant. The holiday season was not excluded except for availability of public libraries opening and closing times. The Texas libraries have cut back hours because of the current economic problems in funding for public libraries in Carrollton, Texas. The researcher took some field notes by hand and computer, depending on the availability of a computer. Hard copies of field notes are stored in a locked filing cabinet along with all other materials that included information that could identify participants.

The emergent themes were categorized by objective content analysis of each research response (Graneheim & Lundman, 2003). Themes Bandura's Social Learning Theory Concepts Definitions Educational Example Comparative Interpretation Confrontation of self. Facing dependency needs is healthy but difficult. Interaction and collaboration as a process of achieving self-management goals. Living with diabetes is not always explainable to self and others

1.
Expectations 2. Observational Learning 3. Behavioral Capability 4. Self-Efficacy 5. Reciprocal Determinism 6.

Diabetic's beliefs about likely results of injecting insulin, counting carbohydrates and checking blood glucose daily. Diabetic's beliefs based on observing other diabetics and/ or visible physical results of desired behavior. Knowledge and skills needed to self-manage diabetes. Confidence in ability to take action and persist in action. Self-confidence in using insulin, counting carbs, checking blood glucose and exercising. Responses to a person's behavior that increase or decrease the chances of recurrent behavior. The use of insulin, balanced diet, exercise and regular testing of blood glucose will result in good self-management of diabetes. Inform the diabetic there is a learning curve, mistakes will happen but efficiency in self-management is possible. Demonstrate how to use insulin, count carbs, check blood glucose and select appropriate exercise. Point out strengths; use persuasion and encouragement. Small steps equal small mistakes. Introduce variable situations such as eating out, hot weather, illness etc. Educate the diabetic to set up personal incentives, rewards, praise.

Positive change occurs with self rewards and negative change occurs with self-criticism etc. Diabetics negotiate, articulate explore and resolve their ambivalence about behavior change when a diagnosis of diabetes is given. Confronted with the daily self-management diabetics naturally adjust their expectations and beliefs about self and being in everyday life. Dependency and independence are negotiable as a diabetic learns how to self-affirm and self-reward progress. This new contract with life is personal and is healthy in learning best practices and adapting what works best for self. The diabetic has a philosophy of self-management whether admitted or not. Doing what you want to do does not work well with any disease.

While perfect collaboration with physicians and perfect blood glucose control are not possible learning what works and interpreting the information to improve the quality of life is always a choice. The self-management of diabetes and living with diabetes is not the same thing. Pity, cynicism, blame and resent are negative reinforcers. Bandura observes that positive self-reward moves living with diabetes to acceptable levels.

The explanation of phenomenon in diabetes experiences is sometimes explainable, sometimes not and sometimes a researchable topic and sometimes not Participant Information Data Analysis Data analysis consisted of the identification and establishment of themes by first recognizing keywords and phrases that appeared to have meaning or emotion related to the experience of adaptation to a systems change. From the systematic analysis of key words and phrases, meaning units emerged. Meaning units clustered based on the relevancy to the research data. A screening was conducted by the researcher asking the potential participant to Affirm they have been diagnosed by a medical doctor that they are a (IDDM) Diabetic person to insure that potential participants are: 1.

An (IDDM) diabetic person between 25 and 75 years of ager with (IDDM) diabetes. Type 1 is the former name used by the ADA for IDDM. 2. Affirm that they are willing to sign a consent form protecting their confidentiality by asking them the questions. 3. Affirm that they understand the researcher's presentation of the research proposal and their volunteer participation in the study by signature. General Deblockedions of Each Participant The following questions were asked of each person: 1.

What are the most important lessons Type I (IDDM) diabetics have learned that have contributed to success in the self-management of diabetes mellitus? 2. What educational experiences are useful in learning about the self-management of Type I (IDDM) diabetes mellitus? Who or what is the most helpful? 3. What have other Type I (IDDM) diabetics reported that is helpful? 4. What has the medical community reported that is helpful? 5. What has the American Diabetes Association reported that is helpful? 6. What spiritual resources have been helpful? 7. What has self-study and self-education contributed? 8. What has been and is most useful to success in managing diabetes mellitus. 9.

What happens when self-management of Type I (IDDM) diabetes is not working or does not bring about the expected results? 10. What goals are essential for Type I (IDDM) diabetes management? 11. What is useful in constructing a Type I (IDDM) diabetes regimen for self-management of diabetes mellitus? 12. What positive strengths are useful that have contributed to success in living with diabetes? 13. What is the most challenging thing that has happened to you as a result of being diabetic? 14. What impact do family, friends, and peers have in diabetic self-management experience? 15.

What is currently useful in improving diabetes self-management? 16. What advice is needed for diabetics experiencing diabetes? 17. Are the experiences of social stigma from being a diabetic significant and, if so, how? 18. What were the most difficult challenges in adapting to being a diabetic and managing the disease? 19. Which support system is the most effective for living with diabetes and how helpful is it? Presentation of the Themes 1. Confrontation of self 2. Facing dependency needs is healthy but difficult 3. Interaction and collaboration as a process of achieving self-management goals 4.

Living with diabetes is not always explainable to self and others Questions The researcher choose a generic qualitative methodology to gain a better understanding of the attitudes and experiences of diabetics as they experienced a significant change in their primary role as self manager.

This model provided the researcher with the ability to ask specific questions about the initial feelings toward the role change and about how those feelings were personally handled during the learning and treatment process The remainder of this chapter will provide a discussion of the themes as they relate to the research questions. Three primary themes initially emerged from the data which were defeat, fear or empowerment... While some of the themes intertwined to address more than one of the research questions, the themes clustered into three primary groups.

The themes of beneficence and capability clustered to answer the first research question about attitudes and experiences, comfort level and systems change clustered to address the emergence of cognitive dissonance and mindset addressed the resolution of cognitive dissonance. Attitudes and Experiences The internal environment is the situation that the participant uses as a self-identity or self-fulfilling prophecy about their ability or fate. These internal characteristics define how they identity with self-management of IDDM. It can also include the disparity between great capability on one hand and disability on the other. It includes denial, organizational struggles, and a sense of difference from others; particularly peers.

Additionally, these characteristics include the need for actively engaging in learning, seeking out stimulation, tenacity, and the benefits that IDDM provides. It is noteworthy that of all the elements influencing the IDDM's ability to learn is a purposeful decision to self-manage with no change regarding new information or adopting new information as an opportunity to have improved health... The internal environment is dependent on their decision they can't or won't do anything different because they will still not be who they once were. It is self-taught or a deeper inability to care for themselves. This is not to minimize the power of the other factors.

It simply brings to light the amount of internal characteristics that these persons have to deal with in order to learn that others without IDDM symptoms would not have, at least not to the same extent. In this way, each of the internal and external environments and responses influenced how well the student diagnosed with IDDM was able to adaptThis chapter integrates all of this information, and observes, organizes and labels the material in an orderly and logical list of themes and insights. Participant interviews with IDDM volunteer participants provided the data for this study. The overall purpose is to examine the impact of the internal efficacy and responses of the participants diagnosed with (IDDM).

The underlying assumptions listed above implicitly guided this study with rigor and a framework as an analytical lens. A non-philosophical approach to what it means to be a human with IDDM guided this study and interpretation of the data. The work of Bandura, (1974), Kanfer, (1975), and Creer, (1976), composes the foundational spark for more qualitative research about the self-management of IDDM.

Research supports the benefits of teaching self-management of diabetes (SMDM), using a high protein low carbohydrate diet in combination with daily exercise, and accurate calculation of diabetic medications as the most effective intervention leading to a better quality of life, and a reduction in the death rate resulting from uncontrolled diabetes mellitus (DM). A review of the literature indicates 76% - 97% of diabetics achieve normal blood sugar control and suffer few comorbidities related to less than optimal control of the disease. An effect size (ES) r using Fisher's Z of the Pearson correlation coefficient indicates in a meta-analyses of 153 studies from 1977 – 1994 "combined Z values more than 5" of clients who complied to a self-management regimen.

Overall, clients that were managing DM by self-management including diabetic education indicated a 100% improvement in the severity of DM and DM comorbidities (Roster, Hall, Merisca, Nordstrom, Cretin, & Svarstad, 1988; Toljamo, & Hentinen, 2001).). The purpose of this project is to integrate the psychological benefits of maintaining diabetic control using a low-carbohydrate high protein diet in association with self-motivational psychotherapy models to encourage persons with diabetes mellitus (DM), to set goals toward euglycemia of 4.5% -5%.

According to the literature, it appears that diabetics who are self-motivated by strictly adhering to a diabetic regimen have better results in maintaining health. Glycosylated hemoglobin semiannual targets of 4.5% - 5% report a significant reduction in the annual death rate of diabetics, and accompanying comorbidities resulting from non-compliance to an effective diabetic regimen (Atkins, 2004; Bernstein, 2005; 2007; Resnicow, DiIorio, Borreli, Hecht, & Ernst 2002; Smith, Heckemeyer, Kratt, & Mason, 1997). DM is an incurable chronic disease requiring management for a lifetime. There are many good models for managing acute short- term illnesses.

This paper proposes that the model used by Dr. R. K. Bernstein is the most effective in controlling blood glucose, avoiding, and reversing comorbidities related to DM. DM is an acute illness that disrupts the psychological and physiological health of individuals for a lifetime. This paper proposes that the American Diabetes Association (ADA) advocates a diabetic regimen resulting in a less positive correlational strength than Bernstein's and other models for controlling DM (Atkins, 2004; Bernstein, 2005; 2007; Resnicow, DiIorio, Borreli, Hecht, & Ernst 2002; Smith, Heckemeyer, Kratt, & Mason, 1997).

The main characteristics of culturally skilled practitioner is to motivate the client to adapt this positive low carbohydrate and with all people regardless of culture. Some of the motivation toward self-management needs to maintain flexibility for all cultures. It is obvious that the human body can benefit from low carbohydrate diets (Atkins, 2004; Bernstein 1(992; 1998; 2005). Best Practices for maintaining psychological and physiological control of Diabetes Mellitus A review of the literature does not reveal a national paradigmatic publication of best practices for treating diabetes.

The American Association of Diabetic Educators, (AADE), publishes an 800-page reference manual and conducts "Core Concept" seminars for the education of diabetic educators. Of the 15,000 registered diabetic educators, not many can attend because of the expense and demands of 21,000,000 diabetics in the United States. According to Dr. Richard Jackson from the Joslin Diabetes Center best practices is a "consensus of ideas" rather than a protocol for physiological and psychological treatment. Jackson reports that newly diagnosed diabetics receive treatment based on the preferences of the hospital.

This is an ineffective eclectic approach harmful and confusing to the diabetic (Tenderich, 2008). DM is an illness that requires ongoing personal work by the diabetic. DM is not a disease that is conducive in promoting physical and psychological well-being without the client putting forth proactive behavior to learn how to cope and manage this incurable disease. In order to lessen the intensity and destructive nature of DM diabetics need awareness and education explaining the negative physiological and psychological impact of out of range blood sugars.

Poor control negatively affects every cell in the human body. A compromise in the health of the brain directly affects the usefulness of the mind producing changes in behavior, personality, and affects the quality of personal, social, and family relationships. The destruction of health also affects the diabetic's ability to work and produce an income (Munhall, 2001). The American Diabetes Association (ADA) and the European Association for the Study of Diabetes (EASD) advocate adding additional oral medications in combination with insulin and amylin to aid in controlling DM.

These two large influential associations are teaching the management of diabetes from a medical supply side paradigm. The historical background of the pathophysiology of DM dates from 500 BC in translations from Egyptian Ebers Papyrus indicating DM occurs because of overindulging in food (Banting, 1869; Bliss, 1984). Insulin was discovered at the University of Toronto during the 1921-22 period. Frederick Banting researching "glycosurea (sugar in the urine)" at the University of Toronto and Charles Best led by John Maclead successfully extracted a pure batch of "islet in" or insulin in 1922.

Lilly Pharmaceutical, in Canada, provided it to the United States because America at that time prohibited the distillation of alcohol necessary to manufacture pure insulin (Bliss, 1984). It is interesting that the first person to receive an injection of insulin in 1922, Leonard Thompson, died 14 years later from influenza and diabetic complications. He was known for not taking good care of his health. Subsequently, Ted Ryder, also a first client lived 70 years using insulin. Elizabeth Hughes, also an original client lived until 1981 and died of coronary heart disease. A low carbohydrate diet was advocated both before and after this discovery (Bliss, 1984).

The low-carbohydrate approach was the modal treatment until the late 1940s when the ADA proposed a higher carbohydrate diet and now includes sugar as part of a DM diet (Bernstein, 2007). The ADA and the EASD do not integrate the DCCT trials of 1993 adequately to promote achievement of euglycemia. The ADA publishes recommended glycosylated levels to the American Medical Association, (AMA), and the American Psychological Association (APA). Their recommendations propose a glycemic level of 7% as acceptable ignoring benefits of "illness work" to achieve long-term levels of 4.5%.

Diabetics need effective models that are easy to understand and are effective in communicating to them the potential to achieve normal blood sugars. The models need to be dual track designs seeking a cure of DM and best practices in managing DM (Arkowitz, Westra, Miller, & Rollnick, 2008; Groeneveld, Petri, Hermanst & Springer, 1998; O'Neill, Westman & Bernstein, 2003 Snyder, & Hirsch, 2008There are approximately 15,000 certified diabetic educator's (CDE's) in the United States with over 21, 000,000 persons suffering with the disease.

The (AADE), states that diabetics do not receive adequate education because it is logistically impossible. Diabetics receive DM education in various qualities of formats ranging from a professional educator to a friend who has DM. Diabetics usually do not search for DM education when they must pay for it "out of pocket (Powers, 1996). A national survey indicates that only 35% receive education about the self-management of diabetes from a class or diabetic educator. Diabetics using insulin (IDDM) received 10% more educational opportunities than non-insulin diabetics (NIDDM).

Friends of diabetics provide approximately 14% of diabetic education to fellow diabetics (Accurso, Bernstein, Dahlqvist, Drazin, Feinman, Fine, et al, 2008; Atkins, 2004; Bernstein, 2004; 2007; Munhall, 2001, Powers, 1996, Wolpert, & Anderson, 2001). The significance of educating persons with DM is a challenge to the medical community to design, and implement a method of education, and motivation that delivers higher results of compliance among diabetics. A large number of diabetics who receive education have difficulty understanding the seriousness of the disease.

They often listen to stories from others whose family member died from DM, creating anxiety, depression, and ambivalence implicating future decisions by the diabetic. Many ignore education or cannot motivate themselves to adhere to a strict regimen resulting in better health until complications develop. There is still hope when complications begin, but sensitivity to change is a challenge for many (Powers, 1996). In an effort to address the crisis, AADE is planning to establish diabetes education units in Wal-Mart, Target, and CVS pharmacies in 2008. A Diabetic Bus travels in North Carolina to educate rural communities about diabetic practices for improving control of the disease.

In January 11, 2006, the New York Times ran an article entitled "In the Treatment Diabetes, Success Often Does Not Pay." This was written in reaction to the Beth Israel Hospital closing the DM education program because of costs, the New York Times made an investigation indicating it is costly to educate diabetics. Education is costly but non-education is more costly (Tenderich, 2008). Diabetic education is more useful if it empowers and awakens diabetics to "practice" self-management that positively affects their health by enabling them to maintain healthy diabetic control.

Providing education without considering the enormous psychological challenge facing the diabetic is not useful. Healthy diabetic control is the ability to maintain glyscosylated hemoglobin as close to 4.5% as possible. Consistent quarterly blood tests that are near 4.5% result in less or no complications from diabetes (Atkins, 2004; Bernstein, 2008). Because there are obstacles that prevent diabetics from receiving empowering, internal locus of control training success is limited. The two most productive models are self-help regimens proposed by R. G. Atkins, and R. K. Bernstein.

Neither advocates the ADA guidelines as healthy or helpful (Atkins, 2004; Bernstein, 2007). Dr. R. G. Atkins' research sought to link obesity and Type 2 DM. Type 2 DM advances through five stages of prediabetic progression; weight gain, insulin resistance, pancreatic instability, elevations of blood sugar, or impaired glucose tolerance. Type I and Type 2 DM are different in that Type 1 can occur at birth or as a juvenile without prediabetic progression. Dr. Atkins' research is against the mainstream medical system in the United States such as the (ADA).

The ADA advocates eating a diet of high percentages of carbohydrates that contribute to the development of DM, and make the disease more difficult to control. His research, and the use of a blood sugar control program seeks to advise all persons by creating awareness of a Type 2 prediabetic condition in order to make dietary changes, and reverse the course of the disease by self-management.

Research indicates that normal control is achievable by avoiding carbohydrates, which is at the core of DM, the inability to metabolize carbohydrates (Atkins, 2004; Bernstein, 2007; Powers, 1996). Deblockedion of the Application The best way to halt the prevalent increases in obesity and diabetes is to change human diets. Carbohydrates produce a pleasurable feeling to our bodies through the brain, but seeking psychological relief from hunger and stress by consuming excess carbohydrates is unhealthy or addictive behavior. Choosing to eat what manufacturers seek to sell to the public is to choose without thinking about the health costs. Change is possible through education and motivation. Setting healthy goals that save lives from DM are worth it (Atkins, 2004; Wainapel, 2000). Dr. R. K.

Bernstein is a physician who has DM with successful management for more than sixty years. His personal experiences grouped together with his medical education led to the founding of a DM clinic in New York for the treatment of DM and DM education. His research parallels the link between obesity, and DM, and supports the prevention of prediabetic symptoms leading to full blown Type 2 DM. He is against the mainstream establishment's methodology for the prevention and treatment of DM.

His 519-page book provides DM education for diabetics to achieve normal or near normal blood sugar levels through self-management by adopting a healthy diet, exercise, and the correct utilization of medication, with frequent evaluations of glycosylated hemoglobin. (Bernstein, 2007) The Diabetes Control and Complications Trial (DCCT), conducted by the National Institute of Diabetes, Digestive, and Kidney Diseases (NIDDK) from 1983 to 1993 indicated for the first time in the history of diabetes the benefits of improving diabetic control. The results were dramatic. The weakness of the DCCT study was not implementing a method of education for persons with DM. Physicians merely handed out material. The DCCT did not emphasize the high cost involved in "not maintaining" better glycemic control.

In reality, costs are higher by not managing diabetes. It is expensive to manage diabetes but it requires effort, education, and commitment by the medical community and the diabetic. Another weakness of the DCCT trials is the low emphasis on the percentage of glycemic reduction possible to achieve. Many have reversed diabetes and have achieved normal levels of blood glucose control (Bernstein, 2007). Multiple injections are more effective in long-term improvement of DM rather than one daily injection, which results in an increase of hypoglycemia and hyperglycemia or the roller coaster effect.

Manufacturer's literature reporting research concerning the efficacy of insulin indicates the proteins in the recombinant insulin do not replicate similarly in all diabetics. Bernstein advocates "correction doses" which is an important concept for diabetics to learn how to calculate for better control and maintain stable blood sugar levels (Bernstein, 2007; Snyder, & Hirsch, 2008). A strength of the DCCT trials is they set in motion a schema for diabetics to "control" their DM.

Control was already an important part of the diabetic regimen but the trials triggered the promotion of "tight control." Labeling diabetics as "foolish" adults or "wicked children" by non-diabetic physicians, and diabetic educators negatively affect diabetics who are unable to attain tight control, and resist or do not understand DM education. Non-diabetic others are unsure of how to understand the "diabetic-self" concept. The stigmatizing of diabetics who do not attain near normal control is psychologically disabling.

Depression and anxiety are often a result of the impact of negative labeling (Broom, Whittaker, 2004Diabetics need to inject insulin or take a pancreatic stimulant medication in order to live. DM increases the risk of high cholesterol, and high blood pressure, and reduces life expectancy. DM education that increases awareness of self-management techniques increases the potential for a diabetic to live a longer, more active and productive life including a higher quality of life. The biography or biographical identity of a diabetic changes when the disease is lived (Atkins, 2004;

Bernstein 2005; 2007; Munhall 2001). In addition to insulin or oral medications for diabetes, other drugs may be useful to reduce complications from DM.

In addition to blood sugar control, blood pressure control in normal ranges 80/120 can further reduce complications by as much as 40%. Blood lipid control can reduce cardio-vascular retinal damage, neuropathy and detect other neural damage (Driesen, Cox, Gonder-Frederick, 1995; Foreyt, & Poston, 1999). The Diabetes Control and Complications Trial (DCCT), conducted by the National Institute of Diabetes and Digestive and Kidney Diseases (NIDDK), started in 1983 as a ten-year study to measure the effects of improved blood sugar levels using intensive treatment. One of the complications of DM is retinopathy.

The researchers were seeking to provide a method to reduce retinopathy 33% but instead found a 75% reduction. Kidney disease was reduced 50%, nerve damage reduced 60%, and cardiovascular disease was reduced 35%. The researchers followed a cohort of 1441 patients for 6.5 years divided into a tight control group after educating the clients about self-management. Outstanding results occurred among some clients reducing their blood sugars to normal. In addition, those who improved their blood sugars for the entire research period decreased their experience of diabetic symptoms.

Another longitudinal study is needed (Diabetes Control and Complications Trial Research Group, 1993). The DCCT is historically one of the most beneficial studies since the discovery of insulin, and the blood glucose-monitoring meter. The published results indicate diabetics can achieve better control and experience less fear from long-term complications.

The weakness of the study was it is not aggressive enough. Researchers determined the best possible regimens with the results they collected. However, diabetics can achieve better health benefits because of the impetus of the research.

Some improved by self-management with little guidance from healthcare managers. Physicians were reluctant to be too aggressive because of the risk of hypoglycemia. Those who were too aggressive experienced hypoglycemia but there were not any fatalities. It was difficult to find a balance with the information collected (Atkins, 2004; Bernstein, 2007; Diabetes Control and Complications Trial Research Group, 1993; Volek, & Feinman, 2005). Understanding a healthy diet is essential in managing the wellness or illness of a person with DM. For diabetics low carbohydrate diets are more important than low fat diets.

This is contrary to the established teachings of the ADA and other groups. Since best practices for self-management of DM do not exist, diabetic clubs and groups rely on the benefits of consensus. Complications of DM are avoidable completely by eating correctly, and self-managing DM by keeping blood sugars at normal or near normal levels. The avoidance of dairy products, grains, fruit, and high glycemic foods combined with exercise contribute to better health for prediabetic and diabetic clients (Bernstein, 2005; Mayers, 2003; Wainapel, 2000).

Parents and others model diets to us as children resulting in positive or negative health outcomes. Change is possible if proper dietary education teaches healthy eating choices. Media advertising, vending machines, and addictive carbohydrate foods subtly suggest unhealthy choices. Learning to choose foods that are not psychologically suggestive through the media, fast food restaurants, and neighborhood convenient stores is a first step. Most people do not understand the proper limits of carbohydrate consumption, and the damage sugar can do to the body (Bernstein, 2005). Treating hypoglycemia with a large dose of carbohydrates is an attempt to raise blood sugar.

Consuming large amounts of sugar or carbohydrates to treat a hypoglycemic attack neutralizes hormones necessary to prevent depression because they are not available. Additionally, when blood sugars are too low or too high the diabetic becomes cognitively impaired to choose the most effective "corrective action" to balance blood sugar to a normal range. A cycle of highs and lows result in triggering a roller-coaster episodic period of mood swings.

Each wave may result in a furtherance of incorrect choices perpetuating emotional problems for the diabetic (Accurso, et al, 2008; Akora, & MacFarlane, 2005; Wainapel, 2000). In humans, euglycemia is approximately (80-120 mg/dl). Mild hypoglycemia is (55-70 mg/dl), and low hypoglycemia is (33-55 mg/dl). Driesen, Cox, Gonder-Frederick & Clark, (1995), report in their research of reaction time (RT) that diabetics cognitively choosing proper corrective action for hypoglycemia vary widely. When hypoglycemia occurs, the brain is not able to store sufficient neural glucose promoting consistent cognitive functions in a stable, normal pattern. This results in cortical-slowing affecting behavior not consistent with the normalcy of the diabetic.

They are frequently given the label, drunk or sleepy. Sometimes anger is a reaction of hypoglycemia. Consequently, social problems are common when DM is not controlled (Volek and Feinman, 2005). The physiological complexities of DM on the human body are a challenge to the psychological outcomes, and variables among diabetics. Knowledge, about DM, intrinsic desire for quality of life, anxiety, and depression are powerful issues that contribute to the ability or inability of diabetics to attempt proactive behavior to manage their disease.

The collection of information concerning the progression of the disease, and record keeping are essential for optimal physical and psychological health. The personal beliefs, perceptions, and attitudes about diabetic control are essential for achieving normal blood sugar levels. Questionnaires and tests are valuable instruments in collecting information for educating and proposing a treatment for a diabetic (Bradley, 1994). Intensive or tight control for type 2 DM may construct a lifestyle free from such symptoms as tiredness, high blood sugars, or anxiety about low blood sugar.

Roller coaster blood sugars contribute to irritability, anger, anxiety, and depression. Poor control results in microvascular complications and damage from non-management. Reversing complications of diabetes is possible with long-term compliant treatment. However, the many factors that necessitate behavioral changes may be risky for the diabetic. Goal setting should include a biological blood sugar target, i.e., 83 mg/dl. Motivation and goal setting imparts empowerment to the diabetic by teaching techniques to control blood sugars versus giving in to the disease resulting in physical impairments, disability, and early death (Wolpert, & Anderson, 2001).

Treatment programs seeking to provide tight glycemic control, and avoid hypoglycemia as well as hyperglycemia are not always successful. The client's lifestyle can become a burden in adopting successful strategies to predict the action of insulin and meal planning. Flexibility and choice are not an option. DM usually controls the client's life when self-management is avoided. Modern methods provide and educate the diabetic with strategies to manage DM in order to provide more freedom, which is psychologically liberating.

Designs using insulin and other medication regimens can be part of the intervention design matching the pattern of the diabetic's lifestyle. This is a psychological benefit reducing depression and anxiety (Wolpert, & Anderson, 2001The promotion of self-management using Motivational Interviewing (MI) is a nonjudgmental method used to assist diabetics "work through their ambivalence" and embrace change. MI is an integration of behavioral change theory, and psychotherapy. The key strategy of MI is to provide viewpoints that decrease ambivalence to change. The intervention advocates maintaining consistent control.

Diabetics are more successful when they incorporate intrinsic motivation to accept adherence to a diabetic regimen as a positive behavioral choice. MI assists diabetics by assisting them to paint a mental picture of the positive and negative outcomes of self-managing DM. MI also advocates assisting the diabetic develop an internal locus of control.

This enables diabetics to take charge of the executive function of their mind and consequently take charge of their DM resulting in less comorbidity, and extending average lifespan avoiding disabilities (Arkowitz, Westra, Miller, & Rollnick,

2008; Atkins, 2004; Bernstein, 2007; O'Neill, Westman & Bernstein, 2003; Smith, Heckemeyer, Kratt & Mason, 1997). Approximately 7% of Type 2 diabetics are able to maintain or arouse sufficient motivation to manage blood sugar levels at a euglycemic level of 4.5% -5%. To continue to achieve a healthy level of care an increasing hyper-vigilance requires learning self-management techniques to manage blood sugars with appropriate diet and exercise regimens.

Increasing interest and motivation for diabetics personally choosing educational designs increases self-management abilities to live, die, or become disabled by diabetes and stimulates positive changes. MI in the treatment of psychological issues arouses a trend for diabetics to reverse their declining health. Confronting the diabetic usually results in defensiveness and negative changes (Atkins, 2004; Bernstein, 2005; 2007; Resnicow, DiIorio, Borrelli, Hecht & Ernst, 2002; Snyder, & Hirsch, 2008). Providing diabetic education, improves the psychological condition of the client when an integration of psychotherapy and measurement assist the client in setting goals. This scenario avoids the physician attempting to control DM and puts the responsibility on the diabetic.

The willingness of the diabetic to set goals toward compliance that are above the 1993 DCCT study targets is essential because the 1993 study accepts 7% as healthy and it is not. A support system is an important component of success in balancing the willingness of the diabetic to choose self-motivation for diabetic improvement (Anderson, Funnell, Butler, Arnold, Fitzgerald, & Feste, 1995). Health related questionnaires can assist the non-diabetic and the diabetic in understanding what motivates their selection of food products.

Making food choices from habits without thinking often results in selecting foods that contribute to health risks. Post diagnostic testing for measuring the quantity and quality of diabetic information benefiting the client is an important part of the intervention design.

A Delphi panel is useful in helping diabetic educators determine where to begin in educating a diabetic about their condition, and the severity of taking care of their health through diet or ignoring the unavoidable health complications, and death from the disease (Bradley, 1994). Anderson, Funnell, Butler, Arnold, Fitzgerald, & Feste, (1995), reported a reduction in glycemic levels for diabetics who completed a six-session "patient empowerment" session encouraging attitude toward client ability to make positive choices using self-management that can positively affect the quality of life, and psychological well-being. Patient empowerment through motivational interviewing is a method of assisting clients with health problems negatively affecting their lives. Psychosocial challenges of living with a chronic disease are difficult to manage without assistance.

The attitude that diabetics bring to life issues affects the successful reduction of glycosylated hemoglobin, and quality of life (Anderson, Funnell, Butler, Arnold, Fitzgerald, & Feste, 1995). MI utilizes goal setting to achieve self-regulating behaviors, and activities to reach and sustain healthy behavioral changes resulting in better glycemic control. Diabetic control and gluconeogenesis requires control through planning and self-motivation on a long-term basis. Persons that believe they have the ability (self-efficacy) to self-regulate their diet, exercise, and medication are more likely to be successful in managing diabetes (Bandura, 1997; Bernstein, 2007).

Persons who do not think they can control problems in their life will have difficulty-managing diabetes. In order to handle the stress of combating the disease with a challenging treatment program the diabetic must arouse a positive mindset. In addition, a diabetic may have such a great sense of their ability to control diabetes that they give up when goal results are disappointing (Bandura, 1997). Effective goal setting is essential in adapting health improvement strategies. Coping strategies for self-doubt and anxiety must be a part of the initial strategy.

Intervention strategies for improvement in disease resulting from using the "medical supply side" fund the development of comorbidities by accepting glycosylated levels above normal as acceptable disease management In effect, society is funding or "medicalising detrimental health habits." Personal responsibility setting goals is a more logical approach for vitality. Setting goals and self-managing lifestyles is "good medicine." Personal willpower cannot change health habits.

Diabetics must self-monitor their health rather than depend on medical professionals to prescribe medicine to enable their poor health habits (Bandura, 1998). Lifestyle habits affect human health as an impairment or loss of "vitality." When lifestyle habits utilize self-management interventions from a tested informed source, positive benefits are experienced. Disease prevention theories affect health including DM. When negative eating and management habits are a part of an individual's lifestyle, they experience the "misery" of changing those habits in order to promote a healthy lifestyle. Controlling positive health habits requires a strong sense of personal ability to accomplish the task.

The greater the self-efficacy a person creates the longer they will be able to control negative health habits. After some success is experienced persons are empowered by their goals, treatment plans and life experiences (Bandura, 1998). Top down care from care providers do not enhance improvement in diabetic self-management as much as patient centered care. Achievable targets for blood sugar control promote rapid change by using a short-step scaffolding method.

This enables positive results in a shorter period when the diabetic can negotiate and seek out flexibility of lifestyle choices without hampering the desired goal (Butler, Peters, & Stott, 1995). Health care professionals may not be as helpful with this model unless the diabetic has sufficient expertise in understanding detailed information required for maintaining self-management on a day-to-day basis. Ignoring diabetes for one day is not an option for a healthy diabetic. Frequent corrections within the pattern of the insulin curve or the physiology of the person are more successful than delaying corrections until an n appointment with a physician.

It can be complex for some persons to grasp and comprehend significantly to manage DM (Butler, Peters, & Stott, 1995There is a "positive, linear function" when the hardest goals are causal in the level of difficulty requiring the most effort from the client to achieve the target goals. When "asked" to do their best clients cannot function if they lack a reference point. Therefore, if the diabetic selects a target such as 83 mg/dl (normal) they are more likely to hit it than not. Without a target, you essentially hit nothing significant except poor control. Approaching the management of diabetes from a psychological viewpoint, most caregivers agree that motivation is critical to self-management.

Diabetics who are more self-efficacious in goal setting are more successful in maintaining control of DM and are empowered to continue to sustain self-care and self-management resulting in positive health outcomes and fewer co-morbid complications in long-term diabetes.

Complications of health, because of diabetes contributes to disabilities and early death (Williams, Rodin, Ryan, Grolnick, & Deci, 1998). Evaluation of Self-management as a Successful Intervention The target population for this project is diabetics who are managing their disease with guidelines proposed by non-diabetics, untrained physicians, non-compliant diabetics and educators who utilize ADA guidelines. Diabetic advisement is commonly a referral of recommendations from the ADA. The preblockedion of ADA guidelines are given without regard to comparison with other more successful programs that have lower rates of comorbidities and a higher success rate of blood sugar control including survival (Totty, 2008). The ADA's recommendation of 130 grams carbohydrates daily is impossible to control with insulin and avoid obesity and complications (Bernstein, 2007). DM results in changes to the body that promotes intuitive introspection to body awareness.

The goal of this project is to create awareness among diabetics that encourages diabetics by communicating they can achieve a better quality of life, live healthier, and longer by taking charge of their diet, exercise, and medication. The diabetic marketplace has sufficient information available to teach a diabetic how to have a better quality of life. Diabetics in metropolitan environments have more access to diabetic education.

Therefore, mailing compact discs, DVDs, podcasts, YouTube, blogs in addition to print materials from diabetic supply companies, pharmacies, and replication of "The Diabetes Bus" are viable options for advancing the promotion of diabetes education and improving the psychological and physiological lives of diabetics (Tooty, 2008; Tenderich, 2008). Carbohydrate restriction has historically been the main model of treating diabetes before Hippocrates until the ADA promulgated high carbohydrate diets in the 1940's (Westman, & Vernon, 2008). The treatment of DM with high carbohydrate diets are resulting in malpractice lawsuits.

Research indicates that by comparison amputation, blindness, kidney disease, and other comorbidities known as the metabolic syndrome are a negative result of high carbohydrate diets (Mayer, 2003; Wainapel, 2000). The target population includes diabetics that have been recommended high carbohydrate diets since the 1940s indicating that high cholesterol, high fat diets was causal as a diagnosis of DM. This theory was debunked. Research today concludes that for diabetics high carbohydrate diets decrease cardiac risk factors. The ADA did not agree to promote self-blood glucose monitoring (BGSM) for 14 years. The ADA continues to recommend, "industrial" doses of insulin which cannot be well managed without complication of DM.

Medicare will not pay for BGSM (Bernstein, 2007). The key strategy to maintain control is to develop and stimulate intrinsic motivational behaviors to adhere to a diabetic regimen. Using MI to resolve ambivalence to plan strategies and arrange personal support systems and strategies for increased control of Type 2 DM increases glycemic control of DM.

This leads to improved psychological health and quality of life (Arkowitz, Westra, Miller, & Rollnick, 2008). The theory of change is useful for diabetics to invest their time and effort in learning methods contributing to a healthier life leading to increased quality of health for self, family, workplace, and society. Using MI leads to healthier habits, aspirations, dreams, feelings, and perceptions focusing toward a sustainable level of euglycemia for a lifetime instead of short-term compliances with diabetic care. The client may need an epiphany or a catastrophe in order to evoke the deep needed wisdom to change life style health habits involving eating, exercise, thinking, and addictions.

Without change, a diabetic will experience "the boiling frog" effect by remaining unaware of nerve damage until it is too late to do anything about their condition (Boyatzis, 2006; Munhall, 2001). Change requires an "investment of energy" in order to reach a level of sustained change. It is human nature for humans to change their minds, thinking and habits. However, the physiology in the case of DM responds to blood glucose control based on the intake of food and medicine combined with exercise and self-management. The ideal self versus reality, in combination with strengths, weaknesses, learning, designs, willingness, and commitment to interventional adjustments is essential for success (Boyatzis, 2006).

The perception of self-confidence and cognitive skills including aptitude are significant indicators towards the success of self-care. In this respect, aptitudes are more important than self-efficacy. It is essential for optimal functioning. Self-determination and the diabetic's voluntary participation in changing diet, exercise, managing medication and, adjusting behavior are the foundation of a successful construct for goal success (Anderson, Funnell, Butler, Arnold, Fitzgerald, & Feste, 1995; Boyatzis, 2006). Complying with goal setting is not easy. Difficult goals may cause reverse effects.

Interventions that provide goals to the client on paper may be out of range for the ability of the "spirit" or aptitude of the person to comply. One technique is for the client to write vigorously about desired goals and modify their approach to what is achievable in small chunks of information. This assists the diabetic advance slowly but surely for a lifetime change rather than a temporary change with a relapse.

Personal and family factors associated with quality of life in adolescents with DM who seek to please the doctor with good blood sugar readings are less successful than diabetics who are autonomous in their choice to self-manage and self-regulate their eating and lifestyle behaviors. This is typical in adolescents who also experience more depression because of not being able to self-regulate DM, and feel inferior to their non-diabetic peers and family members (Bernstein, 2007; Broom, & Whitaker, 2003). The effectiveness of diabetic education may necessarily include an intervention by family members or professional health care providers in order to gain the attention of non-compliant diabetics.

An attempt to empower the diabetic to own responsibility will result in positive lifestyle habits that contribute to health benefits and potential survival. DM contributes to the death of over 200,000 annually and is the seventh leading cause of death in the United States. The significance of self-regulation and self-efficacy to accomplish positive results supports research in multiple studies crossing all socio-economic, racial, and psychological variables. Historically, lower income groups have been more non-compliant and have less favorable access to positive health care when diabetic education is required.

Public education that reaches out to all diabetics is necessary to reduce the cost in healthcare and productiveness for persons with DM. The disease may result from unhealthy eating habits because of unavailable healthy foods, or poverty that contribute to more DM diagnoses each year (Bernstein, 2007; Diabetes Control and Complications Trial Research Group, 1993MI is increasingly successful in assisting people deal with health problems that have psychological implications when related to pathology. MI is effective in reducing ambivalence toward change, encouraging commitment, and advancing knowledge how to acquire the mental energy for change.

Using MI as a pretreatment strategy is the intervention of choice. Pretreatment is more effective in producing cognitive changes in behavior towards self-management. The pretreatment phase of diabetic education may enhance the ability of the diabetic to make changes. Clients who have low motivation to make positive changes toward self-management may need additional cognitive therapy before motivational results are attainable (Arkowitz, Westra, Miller, & Rollnick, 2008; Franken, 2002).

The significance of metabolic control needs national attention through the media, health insurance companies, physicians, diabetic educators, and advertising. Diabetes education needs to be a mandatory part of any diagnosis of diabetes education in elementary, high school, and college health classes to have an impact. Doctors also need training on how to provide effective diabetic education. Giving a client an appointment, a blood test and a bill is not sufficient. Most physicians assume diabetic control is acceptable at rates 200 to 300% over DM recommendation by the DCCT.

High blood sugars affecting the brain are not acceptable (Bernstein, 1992; 1998; 2007; Driesen, Cox, Gonder-Frederick, & Clarke, 1995; Powers, 1996). A significant trend in the 21st century is the gradual increase of a diet up to 60% and 70% of carbohydrate. This high carbohydrate consumption level is potentially a carbohydrate addiction. It is widely known in the medical community that an excessive intake of carbohydrates results in abnormal blood sugars. A consistent bombardment to the endocrine system of humans with consumption of carbohydrates 1000% above the needs of the body weaken and destroy the bodies capability to metabolize carbohydrates.

The pancreas does not have a limitless supply of insulin, and amylin to facilitate the digestion of carbohydrates without anoxerient medication. This is the medical supply side treatment and is detrimental to public health, (Bernstein, 1992; 1998; 2007; Driesen, Cox, Gonder-Frederick, & Clarke, 1995; Powers, 1996). Cognitive behavioral interventional education and personal therapeutic design models are "promising" in helping adolescents, and adults suffering with the inability to achieve consistent euglycemia with a blood sugar range conducive to a consistent level of glucose supply to neurons in the brain.

The ability to cope with anxiety and the diabetic's personal perception of their disease often affects unexplainable behaviors resulting in social and personal problems. The "relative risk" (RR) of experiencing hypoglycemia is influenced by any increase of insulin of 0.1 U/kg per bodily weight correlating with an RR of 1.07.

Therefore, A combination of self-management of diabetes education that includes information about the "physiological wave" response of insulin needs more research in order to assist diabetics balance and correct hyperglycemic readings in order to avoid a corresponding hypoglycemic reaction at the end of the response cycle of the insulin (Hains, Davies, Parton, & Silverman, 2001). Clients that are proactive in requesting diabetic education from educators familiar with MI indicate significant improvement of anger management also. Anger temperament is an indicator of blood sugars outside the euglycemic range of DM. An improvement in trait anger using MI reduces cardiovascular complications, atherosclerosis, and carotid artery problems that are proportionately parallel to the improvement of any improvement of anger. Behavioral research needs more funding and encouragement from diabetic drug companies.

Also important are comparison studies of results based on culture, socioeconomic status, and the ability of the diabetic to be motivated. The client may need anti-depression or anti-anxiety drugs. MI offers the opportunity for diabetics to confront denial of their treatment approach.

Myths, ambivalence to change, and personal perception of success with current self-management of DM are a key design factor (Golden, Williams, Ford, Hsin-Chieh, Sanford, Nieto & Brancati, 2005; Resnicow, Dilorio, Soet, Borrelli, Hecht, & Ernst, 2002). Conclusions and Reflections The successful programs of Atkins and Bernstein in comparison with the ADA and the US Department of Health and Human Services provide statistical research for diabetics desiring a choice between more successful diabetic education models. Collaboration is essential in improving the methods of public and private sector funding of diabetic research. Diabetics with other metabolic diseases than DM require subtle planning differing from clients with DM only. Other diseases affect the need for even more education (Bernstein, 2004; 2008; Powers, 1996).

The Action to Control Cardiovascular Risk in Diabetes (ACCORD) studies are currently in disagreement with the ADA in proposing a diet that denies "normal glucose control" as a potential target. ACCORD reports it is risky and increases cardiovascular risk. The research of Westman & Vernon, (2008), report and provide data that support intensive control. Their research indicates intensive control is not responsible for the increased risk but rather the methodology to obtain tight control.

When large amounts of carbohydrates are treated with high insulin dosages the risk of death from hypoglycemia and cardiovascular reactions are increased (Acurso, et al 2008; Akora, & McFarlane, 2005; Volek, & Feinman, 2005). Since there are no established best practices for treating, diabetes, or educating diabetics, the disease remains one of self-management. Among self-management techniques include the method, and diet of choice. In the 21st century, more physicians and educators are adopting the low carbohydrate regimen. Choices made by diabetics may potentially worsen the management of DM. The "diabetic self" needs correct information in managing DM. The choice of care influences life or death, disability or mobility, psychological problems, health, and progress.

Diabetic education is not simply handing out information to a newly diagnosed client. An intervention using the "Understanding the Model of Self-Care Decision Making" (UMSCDM), is useful (Munhall, 2001). The UMSCDM integrates personal theorizing using other tools for diabetics to make good choices. Persons who are uncertain, may be afraid to make changes on their own. This is an asymptomatic problem because diabetics who are not succeeding with the advice of physicians often internalize their efforts as incorrect.

They do not consider the experience the doctors have with DM or treatment if diabetic education was not a part of their medical degree. Some doctor's merely handout printed material expecting the client to understand it. That is not diabetic education (Munhall, 2001). Realistic goals other than perfection are essential in success with diet, exercise, and management of diabetic treatment regimens. Persons that are easily disappointed because their goals are not attainable as quickly as desired may self-destruct and not regard any positive, high quality goal setting as necessary.

Personal identity as a perfectionist may lead to impulsiveness, depression, and anxiety because diabetes self-management is a life led by blood sugar numbers. Acceptance of imperfection is essential. One track of a health habit or lifestyle will not result in changing all the adaptations a diabetic must incorporate into their identity to be successful in self-managing their disease (Foreyt, & Poston, 1999DM presents hyperglycemia when not controlled by insulin or oral medication leading to death. Approximately 90% of diabetics are obese. High carbohydrate diets and a "sedentary lifestyle" contribute to this problem.

Because comorbidities between DM and obesity exist, it is essential to understand diets adequate to achieve normalization of blood sugars. Lifestyle changes must include BGSM, exercise, and "coping skills" to avoid anxiety and depression. Goal setting and diabetes education are also important. Persons who positively alter their diet and lifestyle increase their quality of life, and benefit from increased cognitive behavior, and skills. Tests indicate that high blood sugars interfere with synaptic efficiency in the brain and interfere with axon potential throughout the body (Foreyt, & Poston, 1999). Diabetics with a perfectionist tendency are also a risk to their health.

Self-efficacy is significant in the diabetic's ability to address issues, and develop problem-solving skills when barriers to goal achievement occur as illness other than DM arise decreasing or complicating the ability to control blood sugars. Hospitalization for other health issues not related to DM can disrupt the diabetic's ability to self-manage unless previous communication with the physician and care team is comprehendible.

In order to cope with change in employment, income, relationships and other emotional issues diabetics need a plan to prevent giving up on previously gained successes. Reaching out for social support is significant. (Heisler, Kieffer, Piette, Vijan & Spencer, 2005). Severe to moderate psychological and learning complications emerge when Insulin-dependent diabetes mellitus (IDDM) is not managed because of clients not receiving much needed diabetes education techniques and prognosis co-morbidity information provided when the individual is diagnosed with diabetes. The disease affects learning, employment, marriage and all psychological relationships with self and society if not managed.

Diabetes Mellitus irreversibly occurs when the pancreas fails to produce insulin and carbohydrate utilization is reduced while lipid and protein utilization is increased. There are many etiologic classifications of IDDM. In order to survive a person with diabetes must take exogenous insulin. The quality of the impact of insulin has improved greatly since the discovery of insulin in the 1920's. The brain depends on approximately 25% of the body's insulin supply.

Learning difficulties, memory, and psychological development can affect the learning abilities of children and adults with diabetes when they are not properly educated on diet, management, and adaptations to avoid hypoglycemia, hypoglycemia, and psychological problems associated with the disease such as anxiety, and depression. Collaborative efforts from parents, teachers, doctors, and co-workers are essential in successful management of diabetes, which is predicted to affect 95% of persons born in the 21st century. In 2005, 21 million people were diagnosed with diabetes with an estimated 6.2 million undiagnosed (Bernstein, 2007).

The Effect of Diabetes on the Psychosocial Development of the Individual Diabetes knowledge cannot be separated from the impact on the medical impact to the body, virtually every cell, from the psychological impact to the individual, learning, and society. Psychological complications develop within 24 to 72 hours upon the onset of diabetes mellitus. Diabetes arouses anxiety when hypoglycemia occurs and depression when untreated or not treated properly.

Diabetes education is important to manage the disease and for children especially infants and adolescents the labeling of the disorder can be destructive resulting in suicide, isolation, withdrawal acting out and permanent personality disorders The advice received by most diabetics in America is probably killing them physically and limiting them psychologically (Bernstein, 2007). The brain does not have the ability to store glucose and thus demands a constant supply from the blood supply system. Insulin dependent diabetes mellitus (IDDM) occurs when the autoimmune system destroys pancreatic beta cells where the hormone insulin is produced. After five years or less amylin is also destroyed. When insulin and amylin are not available, glucose accumulates in the bloodstream and urine preventing the cells of the body from receiving the energy needed to function properly.

Glucose is a primary source of energy for the brain. Exogenous dosages of insulin or insulin and amylin are required to prevent vascular damage to all the organs of the body including the brain. Improper balances of insulin in the body can result in sensation and perception inaccuracies in the brain.

Injected insulin does not perfectly perform as well as naturally produced insulin and persons with diabetes have frequent abnormal levels affecting the function of the brain (Desrocher, & Rovet, 2004). Current studies suggest that cognitive function in persons with IDDM is impaired depending on the number of years attending the disease and the quality of control. With hyperglycemia and hypoglycemia, cognition is affected by microvascular dysfunction. IDDM diminishes flexibility and mental speed when poor glycemic control is experienced (Brands, Biessels, Haan, Kappelle, & Kessels, 2005). Poorer performance on academic tasks among school children is supported when subgroups of children with IDDM and poor glycemic control are compared with IDDM children with good control (Kovacs, Ryan & Obrosky, 1994).

Children were also absent from school more often than non-diabetics as well as an increase in behavioral problems. The most common areas of difference between diabetic children and non-diabetic children were in the areas of fatigue, mood, and lack of compliance. Children with good glycemic control did not indicate poorer academic achievement McCarthy, Lindgren Mengeling, Tsalikian & Engall, 2002). Psychological implication of diabetic control Individual adherence to a diabetic regimen has a psychological impact to the individual and all persons and activities of the diabetic individual.

Well- controlled diabetes may result in less psychological complications such as anxiety, depression and complications from co-morbidities of diabetes that is not optimally controlled. Diabetes mellitus is associated with neuropsychological impairment and effects cognitive skills. Certain regions of the brain are more sensitive to impairment than others. Psychosocial behaviors can be associated with an increase of an increase risk of developing psychological impairments (Ryan, et al, 1991; Gavard, J. A., Lustman, P. J., & Clouse, R. E., 1993).

The work and goals of diabetic educators is not only to prevent the etiology and pathophysiology for medical reasons but to prevent and lessen the psychological implications caused by patients not understand the significance of controlling the disease with available medication, exercise, and diet (Beeny, Dunn, & Turtle, 1988; Beeny, & Dunn, 1990). Clients without sufficient knowledge or diabetes education to manage the disease suffer more psychological problems ranging from learning disabilities in children to cognitive impairment in all stages of life span development increasing with the length of time suffering with diabetes correlated with quality time managing the disease well.

Less education equals an increase in psychological, cognitive, and learning problems in all phases of life. In infants, born or developing diabetes in infancy the psychological impairment and learning problems are more pronounced if the disease is not well managed (Padgett, 1988The management is dependent on the caregiver who must be educated and committed to managing a disease, which will have lifelong psychological effects.

To the non-diabetic and even the diabetic who is not managing the disease well the psychological impairments are subtle and usually over treated with psychotropic drugs rather than addressing the true problem which is a return to a diabetic regimen. Since diabetes affects every cell of the body, the psychological improvement will take time (Padgett, 1988). Etiologic Classification of Diabetes The

American Diabetes association (ADA) recommends that dietary and insulin regimens be tailor made for maximum control. It is somewhat elusive why most diabetics do not follow a regimen designed to promote optimal health and prevent long-term complications. Diabetes is a metabolic disease that is classified as insulin dependent (IDDM) or non-insulin dependent (NIDDM).

If diabetes occurs in early childhood it is considered Type I and has a greater potential to affect the cognitive development of the child. The disease may affect the growth of the size of the child also when reaching adulthood resulting in some psychological adjustments (American Diabetes Association, 2007). The adverse sequelae of diabetes are the result of hyperglycemia over many years. A meta-analysis of 95,000 revealed that diabetes affects every cellular tissue of the body but maybe not the hair.

Diabetic education does a poor job of explaining to diabetics in an effective manner what long term uncontrolled diabetes can do to the cognitive skills, brain, heart, kidneys and other parts of the body. One of the difficulties lies in "doctorspeak." This is the use of scientific vocabulary to teach people without the education to understand this terminology, which is a vast majority of the American population.

For example, if a physician explains that the glycosylation of proteins may irreversibly bind to amino acids and then possibly bind to another amino acid within the same molecule few people are going to understand this (Wainapel, 2000) Millions of diabetics routinely are tested for glycation or "the permanent binding of glucose to blood or body tissues. The singular laboratory test that diabetics should be most interested in is called the "glycosylated hemoglobin" abbreviated "HgbA1c" measure of glycated or "glued" hemoglobin. Diabetes education needs to explain these terms and their significant rather than tell the patient take this insulin and watch what you eat and everything will be all right.

Alternatively, as some diabetics report in qualitative studies, "take this insulin and you won't have many problems for twenty to thirty years." This is incorrect, inaccurate education and treatment (Nordenson, 2006). Hemoglobin is a substance that is inside red blood cells and is essential to carry oxygen to all the other cells of the body, especially the brain. If blood sugar is elevated above the normal range of 83 – 103 the glucose attaches or glycosylates to the molecules of hemoglobin and is carried around and around to the other cells with limited ability to function normally.

In other words glucose glues itself t other molecules and circulates many round trips per day throughout the body limiting the ability of oxygen to do what it is suppose to do, refresh and repair the body providing vitality and energy. Fortunately the cell dies within 120 days and diabetics have a chance to control their diabetes and have fewer of these glued or glycosylated cells floating around doing nothing but damage (Nouwen, Gingras, Talbot, & Bouchard, 1997). The essential part of these sequelae for diabetics to understand is that the more glucose that is in the blood the larger the glued or glycosylated cells become and you have to live with them for 120 days. Furthermore, if the client does not reduce the gluing of these glucose molecules they can expand the next time around.

Large glued molecules circulated through microvascular parts of the brain, the eye, or kidney can damage that organs functionality (Nouwen, Gingras, Talbot, & Bouchard, 1997). The good news about glycosylation is that the binding is reversible if blood sugar is returned to normal limits within 24 hours. Otherwise, they remain glued for 120 days. Educators do not take time to explain that during the four months glued molecules circulating throughout the vascular system they may cause an infarction in the eye rendering you with blindness or limited sight.

One of the most common occurrences is blurry vision because of glycosylated molecules settling in the lens of the eye preventing the eye to foviate clearly (Bernstein, 2007). Therefore, diabetic educators should require HgbA1c test at least three times a year in order to provide information to the client if their regimen is working or not. The vascular system contains some micro-vessels called capillaries 5 – 10 microns is size.

Why don't educators explain what can happen to these small capillaries if a glycosylated molecule is forced through the capillary at the speed of high blood pressure versus low blood pressure multiple times daily for a time of four months. Remember, once glycosylation occurs the human body has to live with it four months and the resulting damage (Bernstein, 2007). Glucose also binds to collagen and results in higher lipid levels, which also are forced through the vascular system and may adhere to the sides of blood vessels preventing enriching blood to get where the body needs it. When this occurs in the brain cognition is diminished, and mental acuity is slower.

Neurons, billions of them in the human body contain an enzyme called "aldose reductase" whose purpose is to convert glucose to "alcohol sorbitol." The sorbitol is then converted by the body to fructose and then leaves the cell. However, with elevated blood sugars it cannot function and absorbs water interrupting the normal function of cells. When these osmotic bursts occur nerve damage can result. Some nerve damage can repair in a few months but some may take years if blood glucose is returned to normal. Diabetic educators fail to teach there are 50 known long-term complications of diabetes that can cause problems in quality of life.

Among these are diminished cognitive ability, ability to learn disability and death (Wainapel, 2000). The psychological effect of diabetes on children and adults In order to learn it is essential that the brain functions biologically in a healthy manner. Persons diagnosed with diabetes may be compromised in their ability to learn if normal blood glucose levels are diminished or exceeded. The non-diabetic maintains "immaculately blood sugar within a range of 80 – 100 mg/dl, (milligrams per deciliter). A deciliter is one-tenth of a liter or approximately 3 ounces of blood. While blood sugars swings occur among diabetics, it is not normal.

Diabetic complication can develop among person with a blood glucose average of 120 mg/dl. Unfortunately in America normal blood glucose ranges are determined as which are the most cost effective to treat. It is far easier to tell a patient they should shoot for 150 mg/dl knowing that damage will occur.

However, most insurance plans and incomes of people do not permit as many exams and visits, especially diabetic education to inform them about the damage a high blood glucose reading causes (Decoster, & Cummings, 2005). For example, if a person eats a large meal and their blood sugar is tested at 140 mg/dl most doctors would not treat it as diabetes because they are so busy treating those with bg readings of 240 mg/dl. While this is truly, diabetes the person will not be diagnosed until the threshold is one day broken and the body cannot bring the sugar down from 200 – 600 mg/dl or higher. It may take a coma to get attention (Snow, & Lawson 2007When a non-diabetic eats a meal, the first bite of food through enzymes in the saliva and the intestines transmit to the pancreas to make insulin to convert the consumed food to energy but maintaining a balanced blood glucose level in the blood stream.

This is called phase I because stored insulin is used. As a person continues to eat, the pancreas makes insulin in response to the food consumed. This is necessary in order to move the glucose into the cells. The body of a non-diabetic then transfers the unneeded insulin to glycogen and stores it in the liver or muscles. When the liver and muscles reach their storage limit, the excess is stored as body fat.

This is "overeating." Then when the person is hungry, the stored glycogen converts to energy by converting to glucose and correct eating habits maintain a perfect balance of stored glycogen and circulating insulin (Bernstein, 2007). For the diabetic "strange biology" occurs. Diabetics have to be taught how their body works and reacts through experimentation to foods and incremental dosages of insulin. For example, diabetic educators do not teach that the liver dumps glycogen into the bloodstream immediately upon waking up. This is a remarkable phenomenon. However, it requires attention by a small injection of insulin upon awakening just to cover waking up before breakfast. All of the intricacies of managing diabetes are what usually discourages diabetics to give up and just get by the best they can.

However, in reality it is possible to achieve normal glycosylated results and avoid long-term complications. Why do educators not know this and why do physicians let it go when they know what is going to happen. Most physicians merely say 90% of my clients do not comply with a diabetic regimen (Johnston-Brooks, Lewis, & Garg, 2002). Psychology and Diabetes One in 800 children have diabetes Johnson, S. B., 1988).

Children are compelled to deal with the psychological issues involved with managing a complicated disease, are not always able to comprehend how to do it, and often defeated in their struggle. A normal life might be lived or experienced without a disease but the psychological implications of a disease that is so difficult to manage without proper education is daunting. Children with early onset of the disease diabetes mellitus present less positive abilities to cope psychologically with the changing world and the demand for learning in order to deal with reality and have hope (McCarthy, Lindgren, Mengeling, Tsalikian & Engvall, 2002). The neuropsychological changes in the brain and the nervous do not have to be permanent is the good news.

However, it does require adherence to a strict diabetic regimen. Not half-compliance or sometimes compliance but ling range compliance. This is a challenge for diabetic educators and psychological educators to impart to clients (McCarthy, Lindgren, Mengeling, Tsalikian & Engvall,

2002). Major psychological changes are made in people lives suffering with diabetes when they gain control of the disease, which may take several years.

This is the difficulty for psychological therapists and diabetic educators to impart to clients; it takes time (Bernstein, 2007). Cognitive deficits are more likely to develop in diabetics who acquire diabetics at a younger age. EEG's administered to children indicated more "anomalies" among those who had suffered a severe episode of hypoglycemia in comparison with those who had not had a hypoglycemic episode. Children in the age range of 2 -5 were affected more than older children. Children who developed diabetes before five years performed more poorly on the Stanford Binet than children who acquired the disease later in adolescence (Ryan, Vega, & Drash, 1985). This is tragic in that with adherence to a diabetic regiment the results would be different.

Deterioration in cognitive function occurs quickly when the developmental process of the brain cannot acquire the building blocks it needs to construct a healthy biological brain. Undiagnosed diabetes contributes to the cognitive function of the child later in life. Research is needed to learn what adaptation the brain makes for neural pathways and connection that were not available during the pre-school years (Gonder-Frederick, Cox, Ritterband, 2002). The psychoeducational characteristics of both children and adolescents are compromised when euglycemia is not understood.

Upon the invention in 1922 of insulin by Banting, it was assumed that people could live normal lives with exogenous insulin. However, the psychoeducational factors requiring clients to understand the delicate balance of diabetes and the chronicity leaves no room for continually living a lifestyle that does not adhere to a low carbohydrate, exercise, monitoring blood sugar levels and calculating the proper dosage of insulin.

Current research indicates that children who experience IDDM early in life develop selective neurocognitive disturbances (Ryan, 1990). Fowler, Johnson, & Atkinson, (1985), and Rovet, Ehrlich, & Hoppe, (1988), researched children indicating a higher incidence of learning disabilities and the need for special needs education. One of the difficulties among young children is the inability to maintain a tight diabetic regimen and properly monitor their condition. It is also stressful for parents who not having diabetes have no concept of what or why problems occur. Most parent assume that the insulin dosage is all there is to managing diabetes not realizing that food intake and energy expenditure has to be equal with the dosage.

Therefore, young children are more likely to suffer hypoglycemia and hyperglycemia not having the will power to refuse sweets at a party or in private. The psychosocial ramifications of such a predicament leave many children with guilt and low self-esteem thinking that they are to blame for the health problem and lack the ability to manage the disease in order to please parents (Rovet, Enrlich & Hoppe, 1988). Diabetes Education and Sharing Psychological Information The quality of glycemic control is essential in the treatment of diabetes mellitus.

The quality of treatment and educational plans for treating the disease do not bring equally successful results. In addition, the quality of instruction used in training diabetics to manage the chronicity of the disease may not always match the cognitive abilities of the client adequately for the client to learn the myriad intricate skills and understand the challenge of managing the disease. The Diabetes Complications and Control Trial (1993) established that diabetic complications could be lessened by improved glycemic control.

The American Diabetes Association (ADA) implemented diabetes education programs to address this need but their results are not as successful as other programs initiated by physicians who actually have diabetes themselves. Dr. Richard K. Bernstein who has lived with diabetes mellitus more than 60 years implemented an education program that continually outperforms the ADA's. His study explores the results of 1) carbohydrate restricted diets, 2) a strict insulin regimen, monitored glucose levels at least four times a day, and 4) regular clinical visits with a physician incorporated with phone calls for help in learning problem solving skills and management of Dr.

Bernstein's study with his associates produced a 27.8% decrease in Hemoglobin tests for glycated hemoglobin using a methodology and diabetic education program surpassing the ADA. Complications from diabetic related control decreased among participants in the United States researched with the DCCT of 1993, and the UK Prospective Study (UKPDS) are both less effective in Bernstein's program. Thus, diabetics learning and adhering to Bernstein's educational program have improved control over the ADA regimen. Nielson (2008), in a study of 44 participants experimented with a low carbohydrate diet.

Low-carbohydrate diets, have an antihyperglycemic effect, are an intrinsic strategy to the management of diabetes. A 20 % carbohydrate diet is more effective than a 55-60 % carbohydrate diet regarding weight and glycemic control in two groups of obese diabetes patients in Nielson's study observed 6 months (Nielson, 2008). The (intervention group, n = 16; controls, n=15) and reported maintenance of these gains after 22 months. The study documents the how changes were maintained in the low-carbohydrate group after 44 months observation time by self-regulation.

Included were the data of two thirds of control patients from the high-carbohydrate diet group that later switched to a low-carbohydrate diet after the initial 6-month observation period. Information regarding cardiovascular performance is reported for both groups. (Nielson, 2008). Nielson's 2008 Model for diabetic control The mean bodyweight at the beginning of the study was 100.6+/-14.7 kg. At six months it was 89.2+/- 14.3 kg. From 6 to 22 months, mean bodyweight increased by 2.7+/- 4.2 kg to an average of 92.0 +/- 14.0 kg. At 44 months average weight increased from the baseline g to 93.1+/- 14.5 kg.

Of the sixteen patients, five retained or reduced bodyweight since the 22-month point and all but one had lower weight at 44 months than at start. The initial mean HbA1c was 8.0 +/- 1.5 %. After 6, 12 and 22 months, HbA1c was 6.1+/- 1.0 %, 7.0 +/- 1.3 % and 6.9 +/- 1.1 % respectively. After 44 months mean HbA1c is 6.8 +/- 1.3 %. Of the 23 patients who have used a low-carbohydrate diet and for whom long-term data, is available two have suffered a cardiovascular event while four of the six controls who never changed diet have suffered several cardiovascular events.

The study reports a 20 – 25% increase in diabetic metabolic control (Nielson, 2008). The initial mean HbA1c in 2003 in the low-carbohydrate group was 8.0 ± 1.5 % (controls: 7.9 ± 1.5 %). At the end of the 6 months study period it was 6.6 ± 1.0 % (controls: 7.3 ± 1.8 %), and after 12 months it was 7.0 ± 1.3 %. It has since remained stable and is 6.8 ± 1.3 % after 44 months. Therefore medication was reduced accordingly Nielson, 2008). Bernstein's Model for diabetic control Bernstein's model of an effective diabetic regimen was chosen because of the results of his study. While the ADA agrees to a tailor made regimen, their requirements are that daily nutrition be made up of at least 50% carbohydrates.

Medical texts agree that when a person has IDDM the pancreas stops making two hormones, insulin, and amylin. The body adapts by utilizing an increased ability to metabolize protein and fats. The normal range for HgbA1c is well above the normal range of about 4.2-4.6 % according to the ADA. They claim that there is no evidence of the long-term safety of low carbohydrate diets. Bernstein's Psychological Behavior Journal Richard K. Bernstein journals his psychological condition experiencing uncontrolled in the late 1940's and 1950's when blood glucose meters and other methods of controlling diabetes were not discovered.

He threw orange juice among other things at his spouse and was not able to function at work or keep a job because of his physical and psychological condition which are inter woven (Bernstein, 2007). He reports that in 1969 his "life was washed out." His life psychologically was turned around upon the invention of a blood glucose monitor, which became available to physicians. Fortunately, his wife was a physician and could order the machine for him at a cost of

$650 in 1969. It was the size of a backpack. Today's product is smaller than a pocket calculator.

This device was important in separating emergency room drunks from diabetics who acted drunk because of uncontrolled diabetes (Bernstein, 2007). The millions who were not able to acquire this information and were suffering needlessly in warehoused psychological units or unable to be productive citizens for their families and society because of their diabetes contrast the significance of this event. Persons with deteriorating bodies were unable to receive help. When insulin was invented by Banting in the 1920's clients were able to come off of starvation diets. The psychological suffering was tremendous.

However, medical problems still complicated their lives and it took years for people to regain a psychological balance. It is significant to consider that 80 – 90 % of persons with diabetics today in 2008 are unaware that they have a psychological problem because they do not follow a diabetic regimen (Bradley, 1994). Data was collected from chart reviews of thirty clients who consumed a maximum of 30 grams of carbohydrates per 24 hour period and self-reported the information on a form labeled as a GlucograF III data sheet prepared by the research team. The subjects followed a strict insulin injection schedule.

The subjects were selected based on an assessment that the client had the ability to comply with the strictness of the regimentation (O'Neill, Westman, & Bernstein 2003). Design to Gain Control for Physical and Psychological Well Being The GlucograF III data sheet is the third revision of a data collection tool developed by Dr. Richard K. Bernstein of

Mamaroneck, NY. The data sheet is designed for the client to record doses of insulin for the day, a personally constructed formula for controlling blood glucose (BG), an abbreviation chart, and a fourteen day input area.

The input area is designed to report the time of day, blood sugar level, medication taken other than insulin, food consumed, and exercise. The form is designed to be folded and carried with the client. A fine pen (0.1 mm) is recommended in the event a large amount of information must be recorded. This is important if the form is faxed to the researchers. A four-page instruction is provided for how to record data sheet information (O'Neill, Westman, & Bernstein 2003). Procedures The participants were evaluated in a 3-day clinical program before the study began.

The study was explained at an outpatient diabetes specialty unit. Upon completion of the three day evaluation and education phase clients proceeded alone. The procedure included a requirement for diabetic participants to adhere to a maximum of 30 grams of carbohydrates within a 24 hour period. Blood glucose was self-administered >4 times per day. Insulin was regulated and all information documented including pre-meal BG, time, and amount of insulin injections and exercise. Follow-up phone contact was allowed to refine the client's regimen.

For the purposes of this study, carbohydrate consumption requirement was 6 grams for breakfast, 12 grams for lunch, and 12 grams for dinner. Sugar or fast acting carbohydrates was not allowed. Clients were limited to three meals per day with no snacks allowed (O'Neill, Westman, & Bernstein Any biological phenomena were correlated with psychological behavior and experience and were required to be reported such as gastroparesis or the dawn phenomenon. Correction dosages made to return the BG to the target range were increments of 1 unit of insulin, such as ¼ etc.

All three daily meals were required to be consumed with a 5-hour interval between meals to avoid crossover effects of previously injected insulin from residual half-life insulin or other physiological effects attenuated by exercise, which included sexual activity. In addition, a 9-hour maximum was required as the longest interval of time between bedtime insulin and injected insulin on arising. Clients were also required to wait 20 minutes after injecting insulin before eating which triggers enzymes immediately (O'Neill, Westman, & Bernstein 2003). An injection of more than seven units was not permitted.

If it was medically necessary, the insulin was to be divided and injected in multiple areas of the body with no single area receiving more than seven units. Hypoglycemia could only be treated with glucose tablets (brand specific) that had a calibrated effect on BG that was predetermined during a 24 hour fast before the trial began. The calibration was calculated based on the weight of the client and 5-minute BG measurements to determine how many glucose tablets were to be used to raise BG to the target level. The purpose of the strictness of limiting hypoglycemic self-treatment was to avoid recording data that could not be supported by the results. Food was not permitted to treat hypoglycemia.

Clients were also to report over eating by measurement using food labels or measuring devices used to prepare portions of food. GlucograF III data sheets were faxed weekly to the researchers to adjust personal formulas for the client's metabolism performance. The thirty clients were selected from person's adhering to this regimen over a 79-month trial.

At the conclusion of the trial Hemoglobin A1c was assessed, as well as weight and fasting liquid profiles (O'Neill, Westman, & Bernstein 2003). Measures The study was measured transversing twelve variables: control variables (age, gender, diabetes duration, pre-trial training), Hemoglobin A1c, lipid profile, daily insulin dosage and weight. Lipids measured were triglycerides, total cholesterol, HDL-C, LDL-C, and cholesterol/HDL ratio. The data for 30 clients was abstracted and entered into a database without identifiers. This data was then transferred to a statistical analysis program (SAS 6.12).

Triglycerides decreased 31.1% (p = 0.005); HDL cholesterol increased 43.3%, p = 0.001); cholesterol ratio decreased by 31.5%, (p =0.001). Mean hemoglobin A1c from 8.4% to 5.8%, (p = 0.002). Type I diabetes had a reduction of insulin from 47.0 to 30.0 units, and type II diabetics from 22.3 to 22.1 units daily, (p = 0.03). Bodyweight decreased by 5.5 kilograms (O'Neill, Westman, & Bernstein 2003). Discussion Other studies suggest a positive correlation between the amount of carbohydrates eaten daily and glycemic control.

This study supports a strict diabetic regimen of 30 grams total intake per day can normalize glycemic control, reduce complications, and improve quality of life including cognitive functioning. The Bernstein trial was more intensive than the 1993 Diabetes Complications and Control Trial, and the UKPDS. Using calculus offers an explanation that carbohydrate reduction reduces the risk of hypoglycemia.

Hypoglycemia results in a roller coaster effect triggered by over consumption of carbohydrates to restore mental stability. However, mental stability does not require a 500% overdose of carbohydrates to achieve balance. Most diabetics behave like this when experiencing hypoglycemia.

Cognitive behavioral training and education about diabetes assists diabetics to comply with a strict regimen and learn to manage negative behavior (O'Neill, Westman, & Bernstein 2003). In a non-diabetic person, insulin is secreted from the pancreas in response to the carbohydrate demands. If carbohydrates are reduced insulin production is less. This logic is productive in calculating the size of insulin injections based on carbohydrates consumed and maintenance of tight glycemic control for maximum health benefits.

Among diabetics, the American Diabetes Association's formula reports less than favorable results because larger amounts of injected insulin are less predictable and uncontrollable during the long-term phase of the physiological response. This translates to a simple formula of small numbers equals small mistakes, large numbers equate to life threatening problems and overweight persons. In addition, correction is more easily accomplished with small adjustments over large injections because of the power of the physiological response in the human in relation to the curve of insulin's effect and absorption.

Bernstein's study supports the theory that mistakes in calculating the correct amount of insulin dosage results in hyperglycemia or hypoglycemia negatively affecting the physical and psychological health of the client (O'Neill, Westman, & Bernstein 2003). Before the discovery of insulin, diabetics were treated with a low-carbohydrate beginning with Elliot P. Joslin and Banting in 1922. The strict diet was limited to protein only with a maximum of 1795 calories daily. After the discovery of insulin, diabetics could increase their daily consumption of carbohydrates.

However, the phenomenon has been one of abuse of carbohydrates whether voluntarily or involuntarily in upward of 82% of diabetics with some studies reflecting 99% abuse. The discovery of insulin led to a longer life but triggered additional health problems associated with over eating (O'Neill, Westman, & Bernstein 2003). The ADA recommends at least 50% of the daily diet for a diabetic include carbohydrates. The ADA restricts fat in spite of the evidence that insulin dependent diabetics metabolize protein and lipids because they cannot metabolize carbohydrates. In the 1920's, before Banting discovered high protein diets were prescribed in order to keep patients alive.

The ADA also advocates using lispro insulin to consume sweets. Research supports fewer complications from a low carbohydrate, higher protein diet with glycemic control achieved by the smallest amounts of insulin achievable. This is modeled by the human body and natural digestion. In conclusion, a strict diabetic regimen requires a strong commitment to improving the quality of life. Diabetics should not attempt this plan without diabetes education that is available but not used by the majority of physicians with diabetic patients (O'Neill, Westman, & Bernstein 2003).

ConclusionsThe psychological suffering that results from a diagnosis of diabetes mellitus is more painful than the co-morbidities and the complications experienced because most diabetics suffer psychologically for generations before experiencing the physical difficulties of the disease. More people die yearly from diabetes than breast cancer and AIDS together, but you would never know that from the level of government spending on research for each of the diseases.

The gimmicks of companies selling diabetes management products, and their message of curing diabetes is extremely untrue and healthcare workers go home, telling their diabetic patients about all the new technologies that can help them manage their condition which equals dollars Bradley, 1994). Diabetes is "big business" linking with powerful economic, social, and political forces without a clue to treatments and cures. Billions of dollars are made from selling products to diabetic clients.

Discovering a cure costs a lot of money, and until there is a cure, there is no product to market, nothing to sell (Bernstein, 2007). At diabetes conferences, healthcare professionals are provided with information about more accurate and simpler blood glucose monitors and insulin delivery systems, but the scientists providing progress reports for curing diabetes, and scientific advances are not present. Diabetes is believed to be a successfully manageable condition by non-diabetics. Many people believe that diabetics will live a full and normal life if they follow a correct diabetic regimen. In reality "diabetes kills one American every three minutes, and every three minutes, four more are diagnosed. Diabetes is the leading cause of blindness, amputation, and kidney failure.

Diabetic complications involve people who hide and people who are managing the disease (Bernstein, 2007; Bradley, 1994). People who are doing well with diabetes, are congratulated and respected for their ability to control their disease, and become the people used in advertisements. The happy face, and not the burden of disease beneath, endorses the philosophy of tolerating, rather than curing, diabetes. For policy makers, philanthropists, employers, and the public to feel compelled to cure diabetes they need to understand that diabetes is costly for society and that those costs are rising, pervasive and the incidence is accelerating, soul-destroying and there is still no cure, and, above all, that diabetes is curable.

Diabetes is one of the oldest, deadliest, and most insidious of diseases (Ryan, Adams, Heath, Grant, & Jacobson, 1991). It is not understood that not every diabetic is diagnosed, not every diabetic has insurance, and not every diabetic has access or knows how to get help from public charity or welfare. While Dr. Bernstein's program is extremely successful it is not available for the low literate, the poor and those that have no access to his books. They are not written on an 8th grade education level. People are suffering and dying from this disease.

Education programs need to be designed for blue-collar, working class, the poor, the multicultural, and diverse among Americans. How many people can participate in 16-week classes to learn how to manage their disease? Syringes, insulin, testing equipment all cost money. The United States is not addressing this disease realistically for the poor and the illiterate. Treatment in the third world is worse (Bradley, 1994). • Diabetes currently affects 246 million people worldwide and is expected to affect 380 million by 2025.

Roller-coaster blood sugars contribute to irritability, anger, anxiety, and depression. Poor control results in microvascular complications from non-management. However, even with these differences, several themes were common in the sample as a whole. The cohort sample were multi-cultural in background, race and religion. Some events did have an impact during the interviews. The interviews took place in a place in a reserved library room as stated in the IRB proposal. In spite of this, the participants showed a great deal of ease and comfort. This was a public and open environment and participants were informed of the choice to withdraw from participation.

There were none that did. Some of the participants needed a restroom break. The rooms were very quiet and comfortable. The Generic method allowed some latitude for the researcher to carry out data analysis. The design's intent was to allow the researcher to compare the findings of Bandura's, social learning theory in application to health modeling and goal setting. The self-efficacy of an IDDM person must be healthy in order to maintain health.

Also, the generic approach allowed the researcher to analyze all of these data within the theoretical framework of learning theory inspired by Gagne's (1985) conditions of learning, Bandura's (2001) social cognitive theory, and Barkley's (1997) theory of executive (self-regulatory) function. or non-compliance utilizing self-management decisions about insulin, food, diet, exercise, physician input, literature and social learning of IDDM self-management. This researcher is not schooled in a research capacity grounded in a philosophic or methodological tradition. As a result the researcher's affiliation is in the self-management of IDDM as personally experienced 40 years, 1971-2011 (Caelli, Ray & Mill, 2003).

The researcher brings the following assumptions to the generic qualitative approach: Diabetes health promotion should begin with goals not means. Self-management is good medicine but cannot be put into an injection or a pill. People are living longer in the 21st century which permits more time for complications to develop with IDDM. "Health habits are not changed by an act of will" (Bandura, 2005). Self-management of IDDM requires a strategy to acquire motivation and self-regulation. Raising the ceiling for personal self-efficacy to self-manage (IDDM). Poor health habits and poor self-management gives medicine encouragement and the diabetic person dysfunctional perceptions of health. Public marketing of pharmaceuticals to reward the disease model should be reversed toward investments in a health model for diabetes. The self-management of diabetes impacts family, friends, peers and the world. The self-management of diabetes is a science for the promotion of health. However, there was still a need for the researcher to practice neutral, professional emotion in order to keep the amount of influence to a minimum.

The researcher took great care to stay as neutral as possible. The researcher began the study advertisement and data collection in the autumn quarter as a graduate student. One further factor was the fact that participant responses came in at varying times. Adding to this variance was the fact that the researcher conducted the pilot study first; followed by a review by Capella University's policy to approve the actual research after the completed pilot study. All of these factors made it impossible to do the interviews quickly. The interviews took place over a span of four months. Appointments were scheduled as soon as possible as convenient to the participant.

The holiday season was not excluded except for availability of public libraries opening and closing times. The Texas libraries have cut back hours because of the current economic problems in funding for public libraries in Carrollton, Texas. The researcher took some field notes by hand and computer, depending on the availability of a computer. Hard copies of field notes are stored in a locked filing cabinet along with all other materials that included information that could identify participants.

Between interviews, the researcher took time to reflect on the interviews and compare them to Bandura's theory. A time of reflection and taking field notes followed interviews. The weeks between the interviews allowed the researcher additional time to think through and reflect on the procedure. After the first interviews, the researcher transcribed recordings in Microsoft Word. The researcher used a Microsoft compatible program (Dropbox), initially and later put into Microsoft Word format. A speech recognition (Dragon Naturally Speaking) program proved to be useful in this process.

After all initial typing and proofreading, the researcher went through all interviews again on the computer, highlighting sections of text that were fitting into themes that were beginning to emerge in the process. During this reading, the researcher recorded by hand the themes that stood out, in order to assist the analysis process, and to cement the information in the researcher's mind. After going over the material and beginning to parcel out the sections that were showing pertinent themes, the researcher took time to read through Bandura's writings about social modeling and learning behavior multiple times in order to become familiar again with the details of his data used by Creer, 2007).

The researcher recorded his findings by hand and highlighted Bandura's theory when used in conjunction with an Asthma experiment by Creer, (1976) in varying colors according to the grid of the learning theory referenced in the literature review. Thus the theory of Bandura and the findings of Creer with Asthma patients were found to be reliable as a model for IDDM themes to the present research according to the author's diagrammatic representation of social learning theory.

The researcher reviewed, analyzed, and color-coded the tranblockedions multiple times according to the social learning theory grid of analysis. From this point, the researcher went back to the interviews as well as the extra artifacts in Microsoft Word. These different Word documents were merged by cut and paste in a unified document according to the physical notes, in preparation for reporting the findings. Once this lengthy process was complete, the researcher felt ready to draw the necessary comparisons and report the findings of the study.

Data and Results of the Analysis The participants all shared stories of struggle that they felt set them apart from most other people, and their own actions and reactions somewhat of a mystery, even to themselves. Part of the intent of this research project was to analyze the responses of persons age 35-75 that are IDDM, and compare the emergent themes with those found through Creer's inquiry with persons handicapped by asthma. The analysis provided themes that are similar to those of Creer's (1976) study. The appendix contains a detailed outline of Creer's (1976) themes. Creer (1976) contended that behavior management for persons with chronic illnesses may effectively be catalyzed with social learning theory (Bandura, 1974; Creer, 1976).

Bandura concludes that ignoring the power of self-reinforcement in self regulation of health behavior is to "disavow a uniquely human capacity" (Bandura, 1974). To do otherwise conditions individuals toward possessing learning bias empowering disability. The results of this study support Bandura's and Creer's results, support Kanfer (1975). Adjustment to managing a chronic illness such as IDDM requires targeting and monitoring self-monitoring and self-observation.

A deliberate commitment to "attend to one's own behavior" is mandatory not a coincidence (Kanfer, 1975). The participants of this study reported similar themes to those in Brice's study in almost every way. They expressed caring about what authorities expected from them and having their self-management hindered by distractions, both internal and external. They also expressed a need to learn independently through one-on-one observation in person or video, such as a DVD and an option to attend classes that were engaging and relevant in person or as a Webinar.

Finally, they stressed the importance of using multiple modalities in the teaching process in order to make learning self-management possible at times. Selection A screening was conducted by the researcher asking the potential participant to affirm they have been diagnosed by a medical doctor that they are a (IDDM) diabetic person to insure that potential participants are: 1. A (IDDM) diabetic person between 25 and 75 years of ager with (IDDM) diabetes.

Type 1 is the former name used by the ADA for IDDM. 2. Affirm that they are willing to sign a consent form protecting their confidentiality by asking them the questions. 3. Affirm that they understand the researcher's presentation of the research proposal and their volunteer participation in the study by signature. General Deblockedions of Each Participant Each participant was an Insulin Dependent Diabetic (IDDM) adult, male or female between the ages of 25 and 70 with and without other co-morbidities interviewed in Dallas, and Carrollton, Texas. The following questions were asked of each person: 1. What are the most important lessons Type I (IDDM) diabetics have learned that have contributed to success in the self-management of diabetes mellitus? 2. What educational experiences are useful in learning about the self-management of Type I (IDDM) diabetes mellitus? Who or what is the most helpful? 3. What have other Type I (IDDM) diabetics reported that is helpful? 4. What has the medical community reported that is helpful? 5. What has the American Diabetes Association reported that is helpful? 6. What spiritual resources have been helpful? 7. What has self-study and self-education contributed? 8. What has been and is most useful to success in managing diabetes mellitus. 9. What happens when self-management of Type I (IDDM) diabetes is not working or does not bring about the expected results? 10. What goals are essential for Type I (IDDM) diabetes management? 11. What is useful in constructing a Type I (IDDM) diabetes regimen for self-management of diabetes mellitus? 12. What positive strengths are useful that have contributed to success in living with diabetes? 13. What is the most challenging thing that has happened to you as a result of being diabetic? 14. What impact do family, friends, and peers have in diabetic self-management experience? 15. What is currently useful in improving diabetes self-management? 16. What advice is needed for diabetics experiencing diabetes? 17. Are the experiences of social stigma from being a diabetic significant and, if so, how? 18. What were the most difficult challenges in adapting to being a diabetic and managing the disease? 19. Which support system is the most effective for living with diabetes and how helpful is it? Participant 1 (P1) P1 was a former medical student and has a graduate degree in Biology. He had retired early because of complications from IDDM. He has endured, heart, kidney, hearing and surgery. Once in his life he was in a diabetic coma. He was found in his apartment, unconscious after 2 days estimated by the participant. He is divorced, recovered from depression and walks with a walker.

He stated: "I would be dead if it were not for Parkland." Through the help of various resource people, reading, and self-observation, he has learned self-management skills that are helping him reach his goals and manage IDDM. However, the researcher noticed that the self-management philosophy is not concordant with some statements such as: "I don't care about my weight anymore." I feel good when my sugar is 180.

Also he passed out often at work and home and started using a wheel chair. This participant has experienced a significant amount of personal and relational stress because of the demands that divorce and distress impacted him. The consequences of those conflicts resulted in defensive activities and significant physical consequences, mainly migraines. These migraines resulted in an extremely high amount of sick days in before he retired "Having diabetes has shortened my career..." I gave up going to school, marriage, and was living alone." P1 indicated that heart problems and kidney surgery had stressfully impacted his decision to retire early.

He blames himself for non-compliance but has improved after recovering from depression and divorce. P1 said that he was so sick at times during work that he would go sleep in his car. Sometimes sympathetic employees would go to his car and check on him and encourage him to see the doctor or health care professional. P1 expressed his awareness of moodiness. He stated over eating was his therapy and sleeping. "Hypo's are a beast. Some really bad. I don't know if I am happy or not. I have been careless and just don't worry about anything anymore. My back hurts a lot at timesP1 stated that he has learned to not be surprised by the misery of hypos but is helpless.

The only think he thought to do was eat sugar. This was at times a physically demanding task. "Several times I have crawled on the floor to find sugar." I would eat whatever, I could reach or find until I either passed out or got better. Once a friend came over when this hypo was going on and they helped me get help." Physicians continually publish that non-compliance rather than concordance is in the behavior of the patient. Some physicians refuse to continue to see diabetics because they think their judgment is the only judgment.

Cognitive behavior is not so easily changed when diabetes is out of control (McLean, 1985). Interventions are not always helpful because a sense of depression and helplessness emerges. Participant 2 (P2) This participant discovered he had diabetes when he began falling asleep at work and falling down by the weight of a backpack. A co-worker who had diabetes called 911 and he was hospitalized. His compliance is now managed by home health visits and a doctor. It appears that a generation gap exists between him and the 21st century and he misunderstands attempts to manage his IDDM. He said: "People confuse me because they all tell me something different about diabetes.

My sugars are all over the place...but I'm ok..." "Each book, doctor or diabetic has a different take on things. It's hard to make sense of it alll." He acknowledged that growing up in an orphanage was a negative experience because the home taught him a lie: "They lied to me and when I got into the Navy I found that out. I don't need God...and the orphanage teachers were strict..." In spite of the limitations that he experiences, he chooses not to avail himself of all of the accommodations available to him.

In his words: "Sometimes the nurse comes in here and throws away all my meat and gets rid of good food. I try to not be here if I see her coming." Adult Senior Services and Meals on Wheels appear to have attempted to help him through church visits. His perception of his situation and choices are noteworthy of analysis. Therefore, he is confused because he does not trust their motives but refuses to tell them. He Said" "When the Mormon women come I take chairs outside and talk with them." P2 is in a chance of life predicament because he lives and depends on aid from Social Security, Food Stamps, Medicare, Meals on Wheels, and Senior Adult Services.

He sometimes runs out of medication and feels that:" I have to do what they say or I might get cut off." Participant 3 (P3)

This participant was Latino and worked as a policeman until diabetes began to interfere with his supervisor's perceptions of his condition. He was transferred to a function within the department that was better for him. He states: "Sometimes I would stare at a wall at work and feel moody for no reason. I carry a Luger and can still pass the range but stress causes me to be confused and that's not good. So I am taking a course in fixin' lawnmowers and am thinking about early retirement.

In 2001 I had heart surgery..." P3 is very personable and realistic, laughs at things he says and appears to be handling, medication and life in general with comfort. He is exploring opportunities for ways to be engaging. "I come here because my daughter works here and checks me out... if I am doin' the right things etc." Participant 4 (P4) P4 indicated that she was afraid of the disease. She said: "I could tell you I am afraid of the disease but I would be lying. I am afraid of it.

My spine, feet and eyes have all surprised me with difficulties." She spent a great deal of time searching out anything that she could find to help her understand managing diabetes but her body did not react the way she thought it should. She blamed herself and eventually sought the help of a psychiatrist. "I resisted the idea of getting help and when I did I didn't want to take the tests. I was not crazy but the tests asked question I could not understand. "But I learned that I could not sit back and wait for help to come to me. It was a very difficult time.

Living with diabetes is very hard". The participant expressed her habit of going "above and beyond what she needed to do, mostly because it was a way of keeping herself from worrying or obsessing too much about self-management.

Participant 5 (P5) P5 is thin and is seemingly compliant with self-management but experiences unusual social symptoms. He lost is drivers license because of passing out in the car with a needle stuck in his arm. Previous to that he hit a street light while driving. He now uses a bicycle. He reports that his lab results are always good but tight control has possibly endangered his life in the past. P5 is compassionate and involved with helping other diabetics.

He reports is is gay and that this has not been a problem for him in managing. His partner is understanding and makes suggestions at times such as eating tuna instead of something else. He indicates that in growing up his mother did not understand diabetes and made too many foods such as pasta, bread, cereal and dessert that were difficult to manage. Over the years he has taught himself through research that the fewer carbohydrates the better. His doctor after leaving home was instructive about changes in managing diabetes.

At one point he suggested an insulin pump that was the size of a backpack and could deliver glucagon and insulin. Glucagon is used when diabetics experience hypoglycemia. P5 chose not to use it. He has managed IDDM over 60 years and remembers pork, beef and the many changes in the development of insulin. P5 said: "A longer life is possible today and I have more flexibility in what I eat. There are more tools to take care of myself." Participant 6 (P6 P6 is in his 50's and appears unhappy with diabetes. He sits with his hand over his eye and under his ear while talking or waiting.

He talks when asked questions but does not offer detailed answers about the impact of IDDM on his life. His father was an epileptic. He still works and when asked about his experience with IDDM said: "Yeah, it's a lot of fun." Participant 7 (P7) P7 bought "Glucose Buddy" a computerized personal trainer and eventually learned computer applications that performed self-management tracking, suggestions, and predictive 90 day Ha1c results. He had an application on an ipod obtained from the ADA that required daily input of calories, exercise, and target blood glucose goals that would predict future Ha1c values based on cumulative information.

He said: "I have calorie food count numbers on foods that work for me. It's a lot of work `but my Ha1c stays between 6.5 and 6.75." The Glucose Buddy application allows the participant to record blood glucose levels and note the time of day—such as "before breakfast" or "during activity." You can view trend graphs, interact in the Glucose Buddy forums, and record insulin injections, exercise, and food eaten. You can also sync your phone to an online account to manage your data on Glucose Buddy's website. An added feature are Webinar's that are available to discuss in a group setting problems and success with managing diabetes.

It can be used on an iPhone, iPod or personal computer and Touch, iPad. P7 said: "Since I input the information as I am managing IDDM or eating the information gives me a coaching type of direction and suggestions about mistakes I am making about my goal. It's like an extra brain." There are several Glucose Meters (I have a Walgreens TrueTrack) that you can purchase a cord for download the software for FREE and it will track all your readings.

I like the Walgreens brand because the test strips are about half the price of some of the others." Participant 8 (P8 did not consider hemself to be normal although he considered himself health. His ability to be spontaneous was rare. The regimen of self management and the constant reminder that all activities had to be planned or incoroirated around the timing of blood glucose levels. At times whis was easy for him but sometimes a surprise. Thus the need to allow control to amndate behavior appeared to be in charge" "I was healthy but now I am not because I have to think about diabetes most of the time. I think my personality has changed 100%.

Letting go causes fear and usually a bad experience with a hypo." Participant 9 (P9) Participant 10 P10) Themes Distilled Through the Present Study Application of the Diagrammatic Representation of Social Cognitive Theory The social cognitive theory (SCT) is recognized as a method to manage health and apply modern tools to self-care. This study recognizes the multidirectional interaction between the potential responses to homeostasis in blood sugar management and the participant's personality and ability to work in concordance or non-compliance with IDDM treatment plans.

The internal environment is the situation that the student walks in with when they enter the learning environment. These internal characteristics can include an application deficit, which is having ability to do a task, but inability to apply the ability. It can also include the disparity between great capability on one hand and disability on the other. It includes distractibility, organizational struggles, and a sense of difference from others; particularly peers.

Additionally, these characteristics include the need for actively engaging in learning, seeking out stimulation, tenacity, and the benefits that IDDM provides. It is noteworthy that of all the elements influencing the IDDM student's ability to learn as shown in Figure 2, the list of internal environment themes is the longest. The internal environment included eight various themes as to what is happening on the inside while external environment has only three themes, and internal and Model of Triadic Reciprocation have one theme. This is not to minimize the power of the other factors.

It simply brings to light the amount of internal characteristics that these students have to deal with in order to learn that others without IDDM symptoms would not have, at least not to the same extent. The post-secondary participants reported that the internal environment was a greater factor in their Model of Triadic Recipocality than many of their teachers believed. The combination of the external learning environment, and the student's internal environment set the stage for the interaction of inward and outward responses. In this way, each of the internal and external environments and responses influenced how well the student diagnosed with IDDM was able to adapt. This chapter integrates all of this information, and observes, organizes and labels the material in an orderly and logical list of themes and insights.

Participant interviews with IDDM volunteer participants provided the data for this study. The overall purpose is to examine the impact of the internal efficacy and responses of the participants diagnosed with (IDDM). The underlying assumptions listed above implicitly guided this study with rigor and a framework as an analytical lens. A non-philosophical approach to what it means to be a human with IDDM guided this study and interpretation of the data.

The work of Bandura, (1974), Kanfer, (1975), and Creer, (1976), composes the foundational spark for more qualitative research about the self-management of IDDM. Chapter 4 begins with a deblockedion of the sample. It then describes how the research process unfolded. Next, an explanation of how the researcher applied the methodological approach to the data analysis is provided. The presentation of the data and results provides a report of the themes discovered through the analysis. It begins with some introductory comments. The researcher provides a general comparison of the present findings to those reported by the American Diabetes Association, and researchers of IDDM listed in the literature review.

Each participant is described with applicable interpretation covered by that particular individual and not the researcher. The researcher discusses the overall themes and put them into the grid and psychological factors of Albert Bandura's social learning theory (Bandura, 1969; 1977; 1986; 1997; 1998; 2003; 2005 & 2007; Creer, 1976; 1997; 2006). This table is used for analyzing these results as compliant or deviant non-compliance of demand side effective self-management of IDDM as neurophysiologic or psychic explanations of disability, pain and dependence (Bandura 2005).

Note: Only 7% of diabetics comply with a 45 point schedule (Segal, 1994). How do those with IDDM learn to avoid symptom substitution that controls non-compliant behavior in the case of self-management? In this section, the author provides a detailed explanation and explication of the themes using quotations and general themes observed by interviewing, recording and studying the participants' responses. At the end of the presentation of data and results, the researcher will describe some unexpected observations and insights that provided important insight, but did not speak directly to the research questions.

This process will then be summarized by all of these organizing themes in order to move on to chapter 5. Throughout the entire research process, the researcher carried out all communications. Others who helped to shape the study's design were the researcher's mentor and committee, Capella University's Internal Review Board (IRB) reviewer, and representatives of the IRB team and Capella University. The researcher authored all advertising materials and then adapted them according to the requirements of the dissertation committee, and Internal Review Board (IRB).

The Parkland Diabetes Clinic, Dallas, Texas then posted the approved IRB poster, approved by Dr. Phillip Raskin, Chair of Biomedicine at the University of Texas Southwestern Medical Center. The subject of this research is a topic that holds great personal and professional interest to the researcher. As a part of having IDDM since 1971, the author's level of understanding of the various components of IDDM, such as its biological basis, its social ramifications, and the other consequences that it causes, expanded and deepened, both personally and academically.

Along with that, a passionate desire to contribute to our knowledge base as well as help IDDM individuals of any age grew stronger. This passion to survive IDDM and flourish and for helping individuals diagnosed with IDDM provides a great deal of energy to study and examine the impact of this diagnosis. However, the researcher is skilled in bracketing and epoche. In recognition of this, the researcher consciously made notes at all stages of the process, including data collection, analysis, and reporting.

References

Accurso, A., Bernstein, R. K., Dahlqvist, A., Draznin, B. Feinman, R. D., Fine, E. J.Vernon, M. C. (2008). Dietary carbohydrate restriction in type 2 diabetes mellitus and metabolic syndrome: Time for a critical appraisal. Nutrition & Metabolism, 5:9. doi:10.1186/1743-7075-5-9

Akora, S. K., & McFarlane, S. I. (2005). The case for low carbohydrate diets in diabetes management. Nutrition & Metabolism, 2:16. doi:10.1186/1743-7075-2-16

American Diabetes Association. (2007). Standards of medical care in diabetes 2007. Diabetes Care, 30 [Supplement 1]. S4-S41. doi:10.2337/dc07-S004.

American Psychological Association. (2002). Ethical principles of psychologists and code of conduct.

Anderson, R. M., Funnell, M. M., Butler, P. M., Arnold, M. S., Fitzgerald, J. T., & Feste, C. C. (1995). Patient empowerment: Results of a randomized controlled trial. Diabetes Care, 18, 943-949. doi: 10.2337/diacare.18.7.943

Arkowitz, H., Westra, H. A., Miller, W. R., & Rollnick, S. (Eds.). (2007). Motivational interviewing in the treatment of psychological problems. New York, NY: Guilford Press.

Atkins, R. G., Vernon, M. C., & Eberstein, J. (2004). Atkins diabetes revolution: The groundbreaking approach to preventing and controlling type 2 diabetes. New York, NY: Harper Collins.

Bandura, A. (1974). Behavior theory and the models of man. *American Psychologist* 29: 859-869.

Bandura, A. (1977). Self-efficacy: Toward a unifying theory of behavioral change. Psychological Review, 84, 191-215.

Bandura, A. (1986). Social foundations of thought & action: A social cognitive theory. Englewood Cliffs, NJ: Prentice-Hall.

Bandura, A. (1997). Self-efficacy: The exercise of control. New York, NY: Freeman.

Bandura, A. (1998). Health promotion from the perspective of social cognitive theory. Psychology and Health, 13, 623-649. DOI: 10.1080/08870449808407422

Bandura, A. (2005). The primacy of self-regulation in health promotion. Applied Psychology: an International Review, 54, 245-254. doi: 10.1111/j.1464-0597.2005.00208.x

Banting, F. G. (1922). Manuscript account of the discovery of insulin, September 1922. Banting Papers. Ontario, Canada: University of Toronto.

Bernstein, R. K. (1992). Effects of low insulin and low carbohydrate on frequency and severity of hypoglycemia. The American Journal of Medicine, 92, 339-340. (PMID: 1546735)

Bernstein, R. K. (1998). U.S. Patent No. 5,716,976. Washington, DC: U.S. Patent and Trademark Office.

Bernstein, R. K. (2005). The diabetes diet: Dr. Bernstein's low-carbohydrate solution. New York, NY: Little Brown.

Bernstein, R. K. (2007). Diabetes solution: The complete guide to achieving normal blood sugars. New York, NY: Little Brown.

Bersoff, D. N. (2003). Ethical conflicts in psychology. (3rd ed.). Washington, DC: American Psychological Association.

Bliss, M. (1982). The discovery of insulin. IL: University of Chicago Press.

Boyatzis, R. E. (2006). An overview of intentional change from a complexity perspective. Journal of Management Development, 25, 607-623. doi:10.1108/02621710610678445

Bradley, C. (Ed.). (1994). Handbook of psychology and diabetes: A guide to psychological measurement in diabetes research and practice. New York, NY: Psychology Press.

Braun, V., & Clarke, V. (2006). Using thematic analysis in psychology. [Electronic Version]. Qualitative Research in Psychology, 3, 77-101. doi:10.1191/1478088706qp063oa

Broom, D., & Whittaker, A. (2003). Controlling diabetes, controlling diabetics: Moral language in the management of diabetes type 2. Social Science & Medicine, 58, 2371-2382. doi:10.1016/j.socscimed.2003.09.002

Butler, C., Peters, J., & Stott, N. (1995). Glycated hemoglobin and metabolic control of diabetes mellitus: External versus locally established clinical targets for primary care. British Medical Journal,. 310, 784-788. (PMCID: PMC2549169)

Caelli, K., Ray, L., & Mill, J. (2003). 'Clear as mud': Toward greater clarity in generic qualitative research. International Journal of Qualitative Methods, 2, 1-13. Article 1.

Campbell, R., Pound, P., Pope, C., Britten, N., Pill, R., Morgan, M., & Donovan, J. (2003). Evaluating meta-ethnography: A synthesis of qualitative research on lay experiences of diabetes and diabetes care. Social Science & Medicine, 56, 671-684.

Colberg, S. R., & Edelman, S. V. (2007). 50 secrets of the longest living people with diabetes. New York, NY: Marlowe.

Creer, T. L. (1997). Psychology of adjustment: An applied approach. Upper Saddle River, NJ: Prentice-Hall.

Creer, T. L., & Christian, W. P. (1976). Chronically ill and handicapped children: Their management and rehabilitation. Champaign, IL: Research Press.

Creer, T. L., & Holroyd, K. A. (2006). Self-management of chronic conditions: the legacy of Sir William Osler. Chronic Illness, 2, 7-14. doi:10.1177/17423953060020010501

Creswell, J. W. (2007). Qualitative inquiry & research design: Choosing among five approaches (2nd ed.). Thousand Oaks, CA: Sage.

Davidson, J. (Ed.). (2000). Clinical diabetes mellitus: A problem-oriented approach. New York, NY: Thieme.

Diabetes Control and Complications Trial Research Group. (1993). The effect of intensive treatment of diabetes on the development and progression of long-term complications in insulin-dependent diabetes mellitus. The New England Journal of Medicine, 329, 977-986. doi:10.1056/ NEJM199309303291401

Driesen, N. R., Cox, D. J., Gonder-Frederick, L., & Clarke, W. (1995). Reaction time impairment in insulin-dependent diabetes: Task complexity, blood glucose levels, and individual differences. Neuropsychology, 9, 246-254.

Dwyer, R.S. (Ed.) Glucose Metabolism in the Brain. International Review of Neurobiology Vol. 51). (2002).

Falvo, D. R., (2004). Effective patient education: A guide to increased compliance. (3rd ed.). Sudbury, MA: Jones and Bartlett.

Foreyt, J. P., & Poston, W. S., II. (1999). The challenge of diet, exercise and lifestyle modification in the management of the obese diabetic patient. [Supplement 7]. International Journal of Obesity and Related Metabolic Disorders, 23, S5-S11. (PMID: 10455465)

Franken, R. E. (2002). Human motivation. Belmont, CA: Wadsworth/Thomson.

Galmer, A. (2008). Diabetes: Biographies of disease. Westport, CT: Greenwood Press.

Golden, S. H., Williams, J. E., Ford, D. E., Yeh, H.-C., Sanford, C. P., Nieto, F. J. Brancati, F. L. (2006). Anger temperament is modestly associated with the risk of type 2 diabetes mellitus: The atherosclerosis risk in communities study. Psychoneuroendocrinology, 31, 325-332. doi:10.1016/j. psyneuen.2005.08.008

Goldiamond, I. (1965). Stuttering and fluency as manipulable operant response classes. In L. Krasner & L. Ullman, (Eds.), Research in behavior modification. New York, NY: Holt, Rinehart, and Winston.

Greenfield, S. A. (Ed). (1996) The Human Mind Explained. Henry Holt & Co., New York, NY.

Groeneveld, Y., Petri, H., Hermans, J., & Springer, M. P., (1999). Relationship between blood glucose level and mortality in type 2 diabetes mellitus: A systematic review. Diabetic Medicine, 16, 2-13. DOI: 10.1046/j.1464-5491.1999.00003.x

Guthrie, D. W., & Guthrie, R., A. (2008). Management of diabetes mellitus: A guide to the pattern approach (6th ed.). New York, NY: Springer.

Hains, A. A., Davies, W. H., Parton, E. & Silverman, A. H. (2001). Brief report: A cognitive behavioral intervention for distressed adolescents with type I diabetes. Journal of Pediatric Psychology, 26, 61-66. doi:10.1093/jpepsy/26.1.61

Hamada, Y.; Kitoh, R.; & Raskin, P. (1993). Association of erythrocyte aldose reductase activity with diabetic complications in type 1 diabetes mellitus. [Electronic Version]. Diabetic Medicine, 10, 33-38. doi:10.1111/j.1464-5491.1993. tb01993.x

Heisler, M., Piette, J. D., Spencer, M., Kieffer, E., & Vijan, S. (2005). The relationship between knowledge of recent HbA1c values and diabetes care understanding and self-management. Diabetes Care, 28, 816-822. doi:10.2337/diacare.28.4.816

Hirsch, J. S. (2006). Cheating destiny: Living with diabetes, America's biggest epidemic. New York, NY: Houghton Mifflin.

Kanfer, F. H. (1975). Self-management methods: In *Helping people change.* (Eds). F. H. Kanfer and A. P. Goldstein. New York: Pergamon Press, pp. 309-355.

Kavanaugh, D. J., Gooley, S., & Wilson, P. H. (1993). Prediction of adherence and control in diabetes. Journal of Behavioral Medicine, 16, 509-522. doi:10.1007/BF00844820

Kelleher, D. (1988). Coming to terms with diabetes: Coping strategies and non-compliance. In R. Anderson, & M. Bury, (Eds.). Living with chronic illness: The experience of patients and their families. London, England: Unwin Hyman.

Kostere, K. & Percy, W. H. (2006). Qualitative research approaches in psychology.

Maclean, H. M. (1991). Patterns of diet related self-care in diabetes. Social Science & Medicine, 32, 689-696. doi:10.1016/0277-9536(91)90148-6

Mayers, D. (2003, July 6). Diabetes diet war. U. S. News & World Report, Health & Medicine Section.

McCaul, K. D., Glasgow, R. E., & Schafer, L. C. (1987). Diabetes regimen behaviors: Predicting adherence. Medical Care, 25, 868-881.

Mendosa, D. (2004, December 16). Books on diabetes.

Merriam, S. B. (2002). Qualitative research in practice: Examples for discussion and analysis. San Francisco, CA: Wiley.

Miller, W. R., & Rollnick, S. (2009). Ten things that motivational interviewing is not. Behavioral and Cognitive Psychotherapy, 37, 129-140.

Morse, J. M. & Richards, L. (2002). Read me first for a user's guide to qualitative methods. Thousand Oaks, CA: Sage.

Munhall, P. L. (2001). (Ed.). Nursing research: A qualitative perspective. (3rd ed.). Sudbury, MA: Jones and Bartlett.

O'Neill, D. F., Westman, E. C., & Bernstein, R. K. (2003). The effects of a low-carbohydrate regimen on glycemic control and serum lipids in diabetes mellitus. Metabolic Syndrome and Related Disorders, 1, 291-298.

Palmiotto, M.J. (2015. (Ed.) Combatting Human Trafficking: A Multi-Disciplinary Approach. Taylor and Francis Group. London, UK.

Peale, N. V. (1996). The power of positive thinking. New York, NY: Prentice-Hall.

Polonsky, W. H. (1999). Diabetes burnout: What to do when you can't take it anymore. Alexandria, VA: American Diabetes Association.

Popper, K. (1999). All life is problem-solving. New York, NY: Routledge.

Powers, M. A. (Ed.). (1996). Handbook of diabetes medical nutrition therapy. Gaithersburg, MD: Aspen.

Resnicow, K., DiIorio, C., Soet, J. E., Borrelli, B., Hecht, J., & Ernst. D. (2002). Motivational interviewing in health promotion: It sounds like something is changing. Health Psychology, 21, 441-451. doi:10.1037/0278-6133.21.5.444

Schoenfeld, A. H. (1992). Learning to think mathematically: Problem solving, metacognition and sense-making in mathematics. In D. Grouws (Ed.), Handbook for research on mathematics teaching and learning (pp. 334-370). New York, NY: MacMillan.

Senécal, C., Nouwen, A., & White, D. (2000). Motivation and dietary self-care in adults with diabetes: Are self-efficacy and autonomous self-regulation complementary or competing constructs. Health Psychology, 19, 452-457. doi: 10.1037/0278-6133.19.5.452

Shipman, K. (2005). The future of Eastfield College: A quantitative study of potential methods to increase retention. Unpublished manuscript, Eastfield College, Mesquite, Texas.

Skinner, B. F. (1953). Science and human behavior. New York, NY: Macmillan.

Smith, D. E., Heckemeyer, C. M., Kratt, P. P., & Mason, D. A. (1997). Motivational interviewing to improve adherence to a behavioral weight-control program for older obese women with NIDDM: A pilot study. Diabetes Care, 20, 52-54. doi: 10.2337/diacare.20.1.52

Snyder, C., & Hirsch, I. B. (2008). Insulin therapy for type 2 diabetes. Getting started. Diabetes Self-Management, 25, 30, 32-33, 35-36.

Sperry, L. (2008). Treatment of chronic medical conditions: Cognitive-behavioral therapy strategies and integrative treatment protocols. Washington, DC: American Psychological Association.

Tattersall, R. (2009). Diabetes: The biography. New York, NY: Oxford University Press.

Taylor, G. W. & Ussher, J. M. (2001). Making sense of S&M: A discourse analytic account. Sexualities, 4, 293–314. doi: 10.1177/136346001004003002

Tenderich, A. (2007, November 15). The crisis in diabetes education: Essential care that's riddled with problems, and what we can do to fix it. [Web site essay].

Thorne, S., Reimer Kirkham, S., & O'Flynn-Magee, K. (2004). The analytic challenge in interpretive description. International Journal of Qualitative Methods, 3(1). Article 1.

Urbina, I. (2006, January 11), in the treatment of diabetes, success often does not pay. New York Times.

U.S. Department of Health and Human Services, Centers for Disease Control and Prevention. (2008). National diabetes fact sheet, 2007.

U.S. Department of Health and Human Services, National Institutes of Health. (1979). The Belmont report: Ethical principles and guidelines for the protection of human subjects of research.

U.S. Department of Health and Human Services, National Institutes of Health. (2008). DCCT and EDIC: The diabetes control and complications trial and follow-up study.

Volek, J. S., & Feinman, R. D. (2005). Carbohydrate restriction improves the features of Metabolic Syndrome. Metabolic Syndrome may be defined by the response to carbohydrate restriction. Nutrition & Metabolism, 2:31. doi: 10.1186/1743-7075-2-31

Wainapel, S. F., & Fast, A. (Eds.). (2003). Alternative medicine and rehabilitation: A guide for practitioners. New York, NY: Demos Medical.

Westman, E. C., & Vernon, M. C. (2008). Has carbohydrate-restriction been forgotten as a treatment for diabetes mellitus? A perspective on the ACCORD study design. Nutrition & Metabolism, 5:10. doi:10.1186/1743-7075-5-10

Williams, G. C., Rodin, G. C., Ryan, R. M., Grolnick, W. S., & Deci, E. L. (1998). Autonomous regulation and long-term medication adherence in adult outpatients. Health Psychology, 17, 269-276. (PMID: 9619477)

Wolpert, H. A., & Anderson, B. J. (2001). Management of diabetes: Are doctors framing the benefits from the wrong perspective? British Medical Journal, 323, 994-996. doi: 10.1136/bmj.323.7319.994

Zimmerman, B. J., & Schunk, D. H. (Eds.). (2001). Self-regulated learning and academic achievement: Theoretical perspectives (2nd ed.). New York, NY: Lawrence Erlbaum.

About the Author

Ken Shipman is an Associate Professor of Psychology at Eastfield College.